Relaxing Into Your Being

Relaxing Into Your Being

BREATHING, CHI & DISSOLVING THE EGO

THE WATER METHOD OF TAOIST MEDITATION
VOLUME 1

Bruce Kumar Frantzis

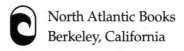

North Atlantic Books
Berkeley, California

Energy Arts, Inc. Publications

Relaxing Into Your Being: Breathing, Chi & Dissolving the Ego
The Water Method of Taoist Meditation, Volume 1

Published by Energy Arts, Inc. Publications, P. O. Box 99, Fairfax, CA 94978

Distributed by North Atlantic Books, P. O. Box 12327, Berkeley, CA 94712

Relaxing Into Your Being is sponsored by the Society for the Study of Native Arts and Sciences, a nonprofit educational corporation whose goals are to develop an educational and crosscultural perspective linking various scientific, social, and artistic fields; to nurture a holistic view of arts, sciences, humanities, and healing; and to publish and distribute literature on the relationship of mind, body, and nature.

Graphics: Michael McKee
Dragons: Jane Launchbury
Cover Design: Jennifer Dunn
Cover Photograph: Copyright © 2001 PhotoDisc, Inc.

Library of Congress Cataloging-in-Publication Data

Frantzis, Bruce Kumar.
   Relaxing into your being / Bruce Kumar Frantzis.
      p.cm. --(The water method of Taoist meditation series; vol. 1)
   Originally published: Fairfax, Calif. : Clarity Press, 1998.
   Includes bibliographical references.
   ISBN 1-55643-407-3 (alk. paper)
   1. Breathing exercises. 2. Meditation -- Taoism. I. Title. II. Series.

RA782 .F73 2001
299'.514435--dc21   2001031213
                                                    CIP

1 2 3 4 5 6 7 8 9 10
Printed in the United States of America

This book is dedicated to the wonder of the Tao

which lets all things come into being,

and to accomplished meditators of all traditions

whose efforts bring light,

balance and compassion into the world,

making it a better place.

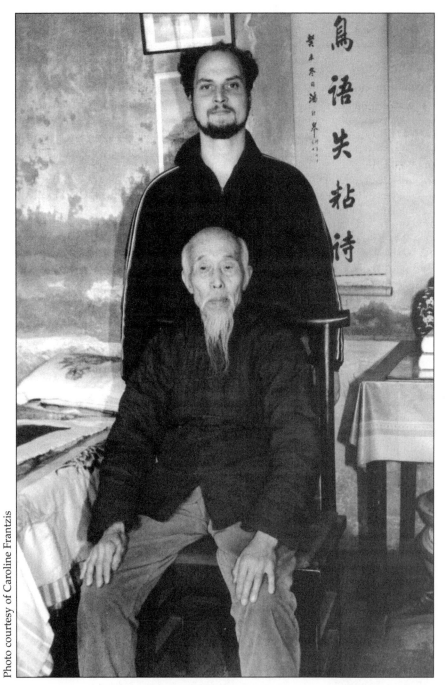

Taoist Lineage Master, Liu Hung Chieh, with his disciple,
B. K. Frantzis, in Beijing, China, 1986.

Acknowledgments

My profound thanks go to all my teachers in the Orient, to the lineage of Taoist masters which stretches back to antiquity, and most especially to the late Liu Hung Chieh. Liu's impact on me cannot be described in words, and without him it would have been impossible for me to learn and share the information presented here.

My gratitude goes to many. First to all my students, whose genuine interest was the motivation for writing this book, and who shared their invaluable insights on how to make this book particularly relevant to Westerners. To all those whose help and suggestions during this work's earlier incarnations made this become a better and more valuable book on Taoism. I especially want to thank those who contributed greatly, but for their own reasons did not wish to be acknowledged by name.

My thanks go to the book's editor Larry Hamberlin, without whom this book would never have been completed. I am also grateful to those who reviewed the manuscript at various stages and gave their input and help, including Frank Allen, David Barbero, Craig Barnes, Brian Cooper, Stephen Josephs, Kamala Joy, Bernard Langan, Dennis Lewis, Joan Pancoe, Eric Peters, Alan Peatfield, Diane Rapaport, and Bill Ryan. I wish to thank Jane Launchbury and Michael McKee for their wonderful artwork.

Special thanks go to the better writer in our family—my wife, Caroline, both for her invaluable editorial input and her extraordinary patience with me and with the disruption to our family life during the whole process of bringing this book into being.

Other Books by Bruce Kumar Frantzis

Opening the Energy Gates of Your Body

The Power of Internal Martial Arts
Combat Secrets of Ba Gua, Tai Chi & Hsing-I

The Great Stillness
Body Awareness, Moving Meditation & Sexual Chi Gung
The Water Method of Taoist Meditation, Volume 2

Note to the Reader:

The meditative arts may carry risks. The educational information in this book is not intended for diagnosis, prescription, determination of function, or treatment of any conditions or diseases or any health disorder whatsoever. The information in this book should not be used as a replacement for prescribed medical care. Individuals with medical, mental or emotional difficulties should consult their health-care provider before doing these practices.

Contents

CHAPTER 3. *Water and Fire:*
Two Methods of Meditation (continued)

CHAPTER 4. *The Teacher-Student Relationship*
in the Fire and Water Approaches   83

CHAPTER 5. *Taoist Meditation: An Overview*   101

Foreword

The fact that this book has found its way into your hands is, in itself, a small miracle. Much worked against it. First, the kind of information this book contains is usually passed only to family members and small circles of devoted disciples. Second, Mao Tse Tung did his best to eradicate all traces of religious and spiritual influence in modern China. Very little was spared, and what remained was nearly impossible for a foreigner to access. Third, the purity of the information in this book is rare. What little Westerners know of Taoist practices generally comes through translations of convoluted instructions obscured in metaphor.

Many in the West know of the philosophy of Taoism through the *Tao Te Ching*. After the Bible it is the single most translated work in human history. In this text, Lao Tse refers not only to how we can approach life, but also to our meditation practice. His philosophy has been called "the watercourse way." Over and over, Lao Tse illustrates his teachings by calling our attention to the properties of water.

> As the soft yield of water cleaves obstinate stone,
> So to yield with life solves the insoluble:
> To yield, I have learned, is to come back again.
> But this unworded lesson,
> This easy example,
> Is lost on men.*

Bruce Kumar Frantzis's remarkable book teaches us the water method of meditation. Its detailed articulation here is unprecedented in the literature on meditation. We learn the difference between the fire and the water methods of Taoism.

*From Witter Bynner *The Way of Life According to Lao Tzu* (Perigree Books/ Berkeley Publishing Group, Berkeley Calif., 1972)

Using the fire methods of Taoism the practitioner forges pathways of energy in the body, using the mind and the breath to amplify or create energetic structures. The tremendous power of the fire method can temporarily override a weakness in the system of the practitioner. Though his initial progress may be rapid, he may encounter limits to his development, limits proscribed by what has remained unhealed.

By contrast, the water method heals us deeply and completely. When all else had failed, it healed the author's broken back. It penetrated to the deepest reaches of his psyche. It led him to experience a profound stillness of mind and set him squarely on his path to the Tao.

The book tells the story of a fortuitous meeting of two men. Master Liu Hung Chieh—a Taoist immortal, classical scholar, and one of the world's great martial artists—meditated and lived in seclusion in Beijing. Had he not dreamed of his coming, Liu never would have considered teaching B. K. Frantzis. Liu had taught only one other disciple since 1949, whom he trained in the fire method. Liu taught B. K. Frantzis the water method of meditation. He also instructed him in the martial arts of hsing-i, Wu style tai chi, and ba gua. A lineage holder in all these arts, Liu formally adopted B. K. Frantzis as his son and passed on the lineage to him.

Having dedicated most of his life to the study of meditation, Chinese medicine, and martial arts, B. K. Frantzis was uniquely prepared to receive this teaching from Liu. Fluent in Chinese and Japanese, this American's encyclopedic knowledge of these subjects accrued from his immense (and probably, from Liu's point of view, relentless) capacity for learning.

If B. K. Frantzis had not possessed a rare combination of qualities—tough enough to withstand the hardships of learning and traveling in China, courageous enough to squarely meet his own physical and psychological pain, and advanced and talented enough as a martial artist to be considered a worthy student by Liu—this book would not exist. This book is one fruit of the relationship between Liu and B. K. Frantzis and a continuation of the generosity Liu extended to him.

The scope of this Water Method of Taoist Meditation Series is ambitious. B. K. Frantzis takes great care to show us how to apply the principles of meditation while standing, sitting, moving, and lying down. He tells us how Lao Tse's principles can guide us in student-teacher relationships. He teaches us how to apply the principles of meditation to martial arts and within the context of sexual relations.

Appropriately for a discourse on the water method, the book moves like a river. Rather than a linear presentation of technique, it draws us through various bends and turns. Anecdotes lead to historical perspectives, to methods of breathing, and to stilling the mind. My advice to the reader is to let the book lead you. Absorb it at your own pace, rather than reading it straight through. Your own experience will tell you where to stop and deepen your understanding through practice. If you approach your study this way you will have already begun the water method, and this book will be your companion for many years to come.

Stephen Josephs
Executive Coach and Business Consultant
35-year practitioner of body/mind disciplines
Wayland, Massachusetts

Introduction

This book presents an age-old system for resolving the essential spiritual difficulties of human life, including those that might seem to be unique to our modern computer age. From the Taoist perspective, our age's spiritual dissonance is a result of a profound disconnection between our bodies, hearts, and souls. The Taoist solution is to reconnect and integrate ourselves, both internally and with our environment.

Oral tradition maintains that Taoism came from the Kunlun Mountains of northern Tibet to China between four thousand and five thousand years ago. Taoism is associated with three prominent texts: the four-thousand-year-old *I Ching* or *Book of Changes*; the writings of Chuang Tzu; and the *Tao Te Ching*, composed twenty-five hundred years ago by Lao Tse. Of Taoism's two major branches, the fire (yang) and water (yin) methods, most texts currently available in the West focus on the fire traditions. *Relaxing into Your Being* is to my knowledge the first to focus on the water method, with an emphasis on the practitioner's viewpoint rather than a purely academic literary analysis. What is contained here comes directly from teachings directly transmitted to me by the Taoist sage Liu Hung Chieh.

Taoism, one of the world's great living spiritual traditions, is only now becoming widely known in the West. If Christianity's central spiritual teaching is to love, and Buddhism's is to practice compassion, then Taoism's is to restore balance in all aspects of our lives, including our physical bodies, our daily affairs, and our relationships to others and the environment. Most importantly, Taoism teaches that through deep relaxation and balance we can reconnect directly to our innermost being—or soul, as we in the West would say—and from there to the source of the universe, which the Chinese call the Tao.

Taoism's teachings for achieving balance may be just what we in the West need right now. We live in a world that is changing at a mind-bending rate. As computers increasingly take over our lives, we all seem to feel our lives accelerate to such limits that we cannot cope. Many people, both successful and struggling, feel overwhelmed and on a treadmill, with no real moral or spiritual continuity in their lives.

Both obvious and subtle factors disconnect us from our bodies. In the agricultural and industrial eras preceding our own information age, both men and women naturally engaged their bodies during the course of a normal work day as they lifted, pulled, walked, and ran, continuously getting things done. Today, for most of us, the economic pressure to use and feel connected to our bodies is all but gone. Labor-saving mechanical devices do both heavy and light lifting and pulling for us. Telephones, fax machines, and e-mail relieve us of the need to leave our chairs to communicate with others. Cars and airplanes transport us without requiring us to use our legs or develop the balance needed for riding a horse.

Continuous daily physical activity provides constant reminders of how one's back is, or is not, connected to one's neck, legs, hips, and arms. Sitting inert for hours using a computer or a telephone does not send the same message. Even everyday appliances that previously weighed one or two pounds now weigh ounces. The more we become dependent on information technology devices, the more we lose connection with our innate sense of how a body should naturally function and feel.

At a more subtle level, we now live in a culture of passive viewers, inundated with a ceaseless array of media images divorced from any sense of felt bodily experience. Television and film create unrealistic expectations about how we should be able to use our bodies, without giving a physical or emotional sense of the ongoing, patient work involved. For example, in films we commonly see a child begin a sport, grow up, and win a world championship, all within the space of an hour or so. Then we wonder why exercising regularly is such a challenging task—one that more and more people find exceeding difficult if not downright impossible to do.

From another perspective, we are all bombarded by scenes of unending violence in TV and movies, from war to action films to seemingly innocuous children's programs. We and our children become inured to this violence and the emotional tone it creates in our society, yet we don't feel the pain of violence, whether emotional or physical. Real pain hurts—it is not just an image—and if we are unfortunate enough to encounter real violence in the real world, we are severely shocked and unprepared for what it does to our bodies and the deeper levels inside our psyches.

Computers also contribute to the process of divorcing our bodies from our minds and spirit, making life for many people a completely cerebral event. The ever-accelerating pace of life in the computer age causes a profound alienation from ourselves, others, and nature. The human body is a precious thing, something more than disembodied bytes of information in a databank. Just as humans were constantly comparing their bodies with machines during the Industrial Revolution, so are people misidentifying their bodies with computers in the new information revolution. An extreme example of misidentification is the preoccupation with cyber-sex on the Internet, where a live, vibrant, physical, emotional, and psychic experience is turned into a dead simulation that teaches us that we are not human beings with living spirits but are merely disembodied images.

Today, in our era of rampant overpopulation, cultural change, and amorality, it is easy to disconnect from our hearts and souls. Societal expectations of what we ought to do, say, and feel, along with the public images we feel we should project, are often at odds with our deeper honest feelings and spiritual aspirations. With severe economic competition, and with so much to do and so little time in which to do it, people commonly perceive that they have no time for deep personal relationships, prayer, deep reflection, or meditation. Yet these are the soil that allows our true spirituality to grow. If we can't be honest and open to what we genuinely feel within ourselves, how can we hope to connect to our spirit, which is intrinsically honest and open?

All great spiritual traditions have at their core great truths and ways of living that transcend time. Despite its antiquity, the Taoist water tradition is singularly relevant to the needs of the computer age. It helps people resolve and come to terms with many of the human condition's basic spiritual questions:

- Why am I here?
- What is the nature of spirituality?
- How can I overcome the conditionings of child-hood and become emotionally and spiritually mature?
- How can I resolve my spiritual, psychic, and emotional pain?
- How can I come to terms with death and dying?
- How can I remove the obstacles to change, come to accept myself as a worthy human being, and learn to live a balanced life that leaves me personally satisfied and in harmony with those around me?

These central questions have been addressed by all of the world's great spiritual traditions. Within each of those traditions one may discern two fundamentally different ways in which individuals have sought answers to them. The first follows the outer path of organized, belief-centered religion. The second follows the inner path of direct internal spiritual experience, or what are commonly called the mystic or esoteric spiritual traditions.

Examples of belief-centered religions both East and West include Christianity, Judaism, Islam, Hinduism, Buddhism, and the external Taoist religion called *tao jiao*. At the core of these organized religions are several basic ideas held in common. They all require faith in the existence of an external supreme spiritual being or beings. You and God (or the gods) are intrinsically separate and different. God rules and controls your fate in the afterlife. Many traditions assert that you cannot personally know God until after you are dead. The religious establishment is the intermediary between you and God. All these factors may put a person in direct conflict between rationality on the one hand and faith on the other.

Each organized outer tradition usually has its parallel inner mystic spiritual tradition. Christianity has Gnosticism; Judaism has the Kaballah; Islam has Sufism; Hinduism has yoga and Hindu tantra; Buddhism has Zen, Tibetan tantra, and the Dzogchen tradition; and Taoism has Taoist meditation. The inner mystic traditions are also based on several basic ideas held in common. They require faith that a human can directly connect at the center of his or her heart and mind to the permanent unnameable Consciousness, which exists forever and, like the burning bush Moses encountered, does not consume itself. God does not exist outside of you; rather, as the Gnostic Christian tradition believes, the kingdom of God is within. However, to maintain a consistent, direct experience of the unchanging root of the universe as a continuous living awareness, without anyone in the middle, requires you to expend tremendous effort to truly go into, clear out, and reintegrate with the depths of your being.

In organized outer religions, people often experience peak spiritual experiences during intensely focused prayer. In so doing, they participate in meditation without labeling it as such. Prayer (mantras) and contemplation are also used as vehicles in the mystic traditions for going inside and finding God, regardless of the specific ideas, mental states and meanings behind what they are doing.

Some of the qualities that identify a prophet or saint are that person's direct visions of God and experiences of religious ecstasy. In modern times we call these moments "peak experiences," as they are above and beyond the realm of normal life. These peak experiences are usually labeled as having a divine origin. In the inner mystic methods that are not centered on belief in a deity, people also reach this same quality of spiritual epiphany, purely by practicing methods of meditation. In both cases the individual focuses all of his or her energies and progressively goes deeper and deeper inside, ultimately penetrating to the deepest recesses of the self, where visions, religious ecstasy, and integration are a normal part of God's kingdom within. It is the act of paying concentrated attention to the deepest realms of the heart that opens up the inner world.

All the inner traditions, which have stood the test of time for thousands of years, have precise and systematic methodologies for going into the heart of human consciousness. The Taoist water method of meditation has its own set of techniques, which are the subject of this book.

People engage in Taoist spiritual work for three primary reasons. The first is the need to cope with the ever-increasing pressures of the computerized age, including civilization's stresses on our physical, emotional, and mental health. The resolution to those pressures is found in the preparatory practices described in this volume, exercises in which you energize, heal, and relax the body as you simultaneously slow down, quiet, and release the tensions within the mind.

The second reason is a desire to connect directly and in a deeply personal way to an ever-present source of spirituality that is greater than our limited personality and ego. This source is what we in the West call the soul, and what the Taoists call *being*. The resolution to this primal need is found in the Taoist meditation practices explained herein, practices in which you learn to dissolve and resolve the inner spiritual, emotional, and psychic conflicts that prevent your mind and spirit from becoming still. From that place of stillness you come to experience great inner peace.

The third reason is the spiritual need to transform your inner world until your individuality directly merges with the unchanging source of the universe—what in different times and places has been called by many names, including God, Spirit, a Higher Power, Universal Consciousness, and the Tao. The resolution of this need is found in the exceedingly challenging Taoist inner alchemy practices, which ultimately result in what various traditions describe as enlightenment, union with God, or the Buddha mind. This stage of meditation, which is introduced in volume 2 of this

Water Method of Taoist Meditation Series, *The Great Stillness*, requires an open-ended commitment for as much time as it takes, be it years, decades, or lives.

The process of Taoist meditation is circular rather than linear; that is, it is not a simple matter of mastering one thing and then moving on to the next. The learning process is like an ever-continuing spiral of self-exploration. As you move from one round of learning to the next, two things occur simultaneously: (1) you learn something new, and (2) you relearn previous material at a greater depth. The latter occurs not only because more information is directly stated but also because deeper levels of your mind have been prepared and opened, allowing you to experience more completely aspects of the Tao that can be indirectly hinted at but not overtly said. Often these insights will come upon you suddenly, although exactly why, when, and how will be hard to say.

This circular quality is reflected in the nonlinear structure of this book. In the first pass around the circle, chapters 1 through 4 give a pragmatic overview of the vibrant living spiritual tradition of Taoism, rather than its dry academic, philosophical, or literary aspects. These four chapters show how Taoist practices can benefit people regardless of formal religious affiliation. The common points and differences between the two main branches of Taoism, the fire and water methods, are explored, both in terms of how and why they use various spiritual and energetic practices, and in terms of the teaching approaches each method takes. Chapter 4 in particular addresses the teacher-student relationship, an aspect of spiritual traditions that has been much abused in recent years, especially in the West. Throughout these chapters the reader is introduced to the first lessons in Taoist internal breathing, which is the foundation of all the meditation practices described in this volume and the next in the series. These techniques will both increase your breathing capacity, benefit your health, and allow your awareness to feel and experience the energies within your body.

In the second pass around the circle, chapters 5 through 8 describe in detail the benefits, goals, and practice methods of the preparatory and intermediate stages of Taoist meditation. Chapters 5 and 6 describe practices, in the standing and moving modes respectively, that open the body's energy channels and promote physical health, mental relaxation, and a stable awareness of the internal workings of your body and mind. These practices also create an environment in which may occur the "wonderful accident," wherein you stumble upon a flash of spiritual insight and directly glimpse the Universal Consciousness that resides within us all.

These beginning practices primarily work with the physical and energetic aspects of the human mind and body, and not the deeper emotional and psychic aspects, which are the primary concern of Chapters 7 and 8. These beginning practices lay the foundation for the latter chapters' deeper intermediate meditation practices for stilling the mind and directly connecting to Universal Consciousness. This foundation is strengthened with the completion of the Taoist internal breathing lessons begun in the earlier chapters.

Chapters 7 and 8 focus on the intermediate stage of Taoist meditation. Here the techniques for releasing the energies of a human's deepest inner emotional, mental, psychic, and spiritual blockages are explored fully. During this stage you learn to resolve your own inner demons, as well as develop and mature your spirituality, as the deepest layers of your energies and mind gradually become smooth and quiet. Eventually, when the mind settles sufficiently, the meditator begins to realize the emptiness of the mind in stages, until the mind becomes completely still. At this point the Universal Consciousness becomes apparent and ever present in your normal awareness. You become like a newly born spiritual infant, continuously aware of the all-pervading Consciousness that is both within you and all around you. This awareness naturally creates a stable spiritual center within, so you never again feel disconnected from a profound, personally felt source of living spirituality.

After thoroughly assimilating the material in this first volume, the reader will be ready to explore the more advanced techniques in volume 2, *The Great Stillness*, which includes additional practices in the standing and moving modes as well as those done sitting, lying down, and during sexual activity. The second volume also offers an introduction to Taoist internal alchemy. Most importantly, it explores in greater depth the inner dissolving process, the central technique of the intermediate practices. It must be remembered, however, that work done at the more advanced stages will be of value only if a proper foundation has been laid in the preparatory and intermediate stages detailed in volume 1.

The first appendix to the present volume answers several questions commonly asked by practitioners of Taoist meditation and of meditation in general. The second illustrates the main energy channels and centers of the human body.

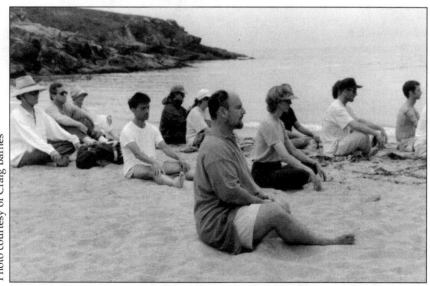

Photo courtesy of Craig Barnes

Frantzis leads a meditation retreat in Northern California.

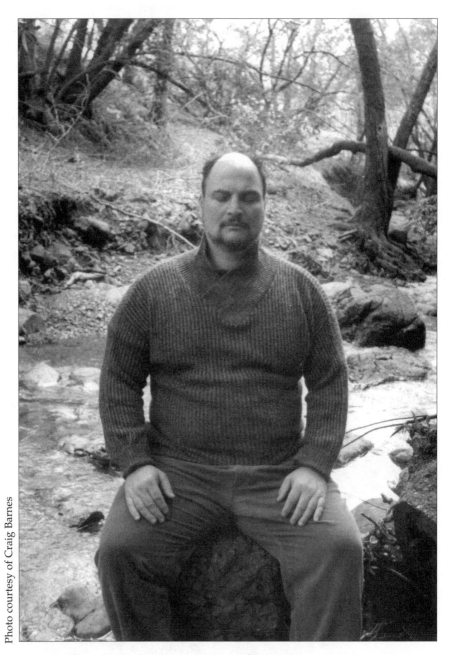

The author, B. K. Frantzis, in meditation.

Connecting with Chi

CHAPTER 1

Chuang Tzu Being Whole

The qualities of Nature sink to their roots in the Tao
The secrets of our vital force and power
Are protected and hidden within the Tao

Connecting with Chi

The Taoist Tradition

In the Western world, Taoism is known primarily through certain of its pragmatic arts. The Taoist martial arts, such as tai chi, are getting more exposure; the stress reduction and medical aspects of chi gung are gaining attention; Chinese medicine (another Taoist art) is attracting wider interest; even geomancy (*feng shui*)—analyzing energy patterns by means of interior spatial or geographical features—is becoming familiar. Taoist meditation, however, is much less known in the West.

The Taoist canon, which consists of over a thousand books, includes the topic of meditation, but the canon has not been completely translated into English. In fact, the world outside China has not seen anywhere near the bulk of it yet. Moreover, the few books that exist in English have mostly been translated by scholars rather than by practitioners. As a result, many important concepts and words have been misconstrued in translation. Their literal meanings have been substituted for their actual intent, flavor, and deeper significance, thus distorting the picture they present. The chart on page 30 serves to show what has been derived from Taoist meditation—its family tree, as it were.

Practices Derived from Taoist Meditation

Diagram A

WHAT HAS ORIGINATED FROM TAOIST MEDITATION: A LINEAGE

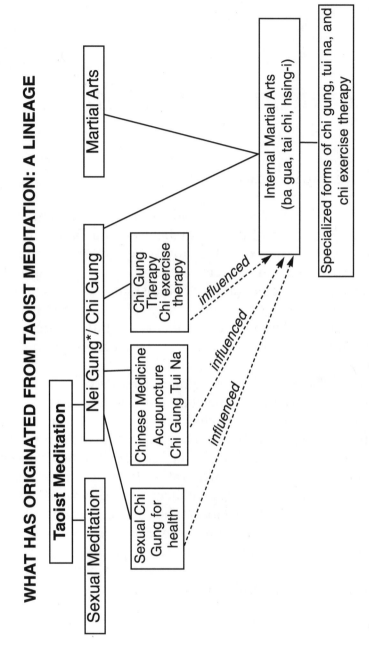

*Nei gung refers to the development of internal power; chi gung to internal energy work.

About the Word *Chi*

The word *chi* is bandied about freely in English. It is most often taken to be the equivalent of the word *energy* and can be applied to anything, as everything that exists is a form of energy (the chi of this or that, protective chi, pre-birth chi, etc.). This book, however, uses the word chi a bit more carefully in order to differentiate contexts.

In Chinese medicine, *chi* refers to the energy that causes the physical body to function (that which allows you to move, speak, and so on). The chi of Chinese medicine is the equivalent of the first and second energy bodies of the Taoists (the chi body), which refers to our physical anatomy and the energy that makes it alive. (See pp. 50–54 for a complete description of the Taoist system of the energetic levels or "bodies.") When it is used in this context, chi will be spelled with a lowercase *c*.

In addition to this chi of Chinese medicine (or second-body chi), the Taoists apply yet another spiritual meaning to this word. In Taoist meditation, the concept "chi" refers specifically to what the Taoists identify as the third, fourth, fifth, and sixth energetic levels or "bodies" of human beings. The third energetic level is the emotional body, the power that allows for the higher emotions. The fourth energetic level is the mental body, the power that fuels concrete thought. The fifth and sixth energetic bodies are normally referred to as *shen*, or spirit. The fifth energetic level is the psychic energy body, through which we find our hidden internal capacities. The sixth energetic level, or causal body, is related to time and space. All of these energies (the first through sixth bodies) form the context represented by spelling Chi with a capital *C*—that is, both physical and nonphysical energies viewed as a continuum. This is also the Chi and Spirit of the Three Treasures (see p. 56).

To avoid confusion, when we speak herein of general energy, we will use the word *energy* and not the word *chi*.

FOCUS ON PRACTICE
How to Tell the Difference between Feeling Physical Sensations and Feeling Chi

 Both your physical body and chi generate sensations you can feel. The sensation of chi is just as concrete as the physical body, only slightly more subtle, with a feeling that is lighter, noncorporeal, but nonetheless very real. Some compare it to bioelectricity. Electric current has a more subtle feeling than physical matter yet has a distinct range of sensations. Some of the standard sensations of chi are heat, cold, pressure, wind, light, electricity, numbness, and mist.

One traditional way to distinguish between physicality and chi is to experience the difference between the physical and energetic sensations of your palms. The palms are the easiest place to feel chi in the body. First rub your palms together and concentrate on the physical feeling evoked. Next, put your palms four or five inches apart, with the centers of your palms facing each other. Close your eyes. Move your palms around (with their centers always facing each other) until you feel a small ball of energy between them, or you can feel some kind of energy or pressure connecting them. These are the sensations of chi. Next rub your hands together and again compare the two feelings: physicality and chi.

Another way is to observe the kind of sensations that sexual energy generates within you. During sexual contact, your Chi takes on a specific frequency that you experience as sexual energy. In fact, sexual energy is simply one variation of the life force. There are other types of chi whose sensations are just as strong or as weak, whichever the case may be. Some people may experience nonsexual forms of chi as stronger or weaker than sexual energy itself. However, the nonsexual forms of chi do not a have a sexual charge. They feel different from sexual energy because they vibrate at different frequencies, some quite strong and some neutral. In the whole gamut of Chi, or life force energy, sexual energy is but one kind.

In a platonic relationship, a touching of hands or a peck on the cheek is usually a fairly physical experience. In a sexual context however, a touch or kiss can send an energy wave within and throughout one or both of the participant's bodies. This wave is chi.

What Is Taoist Meditation?

Who am I? What does it mean to be human and fully alive? What is my relationship to the vastness of eternity? How can I find inner comfort in the stressful, swirling circumstances of life? How can I reconcile the physical needs of having a body with being spiritual?

Using meditation, Taoists have sought useful and heartfelt answers to these kinds of primal questions for over five thousand years. The living tradition of Taoist meditation has sought from its inception to balance the realities of the human condition—that is, our having to live with a temporary physical body while simultaneously establishing contact with a permanent, personally experienced spiritual center. Taoist meditation is about several things. First, it provides us with practical means to enhance the physical, emotional, mental, and psychic parts of ourselves. Second, it allows an individual to be comfortably at home in mind, spirit, and an ever-changing physical body. Third, it enables us with our normal, everyday consciousness to experience a direct, personal connection with the always present and never-ending Universal Consciousness from which all phenomena arise.*

Learning Taoist Meditation

To learn Taoist meditation properly, a student should start with certain preparatory (beginning) practices, then progress through intermediate (middle) to concluding (advanced) practices. This book explains the preparatory and intermediate practices. Volume 2 of this Water Method of Taoist Meditation Series, *The Great Stillness*, contains more advanced practices. The diagrams on pages 34, 35, and 36 serve as basic guides to which activities take place at each

---

*Throughout this book, mundane consciousness is spelled with a small *c*, Universal Consciousness with a capital C.

Preparatory (Beginning) Practices

The aim of the beginning practices is to develop an awareness of subtle energy in your body and to maintain that awareness. The benefits of the beginning practices include improved health, vitality, calmness, and the awareness necessary for the middle practices.

Diagram B

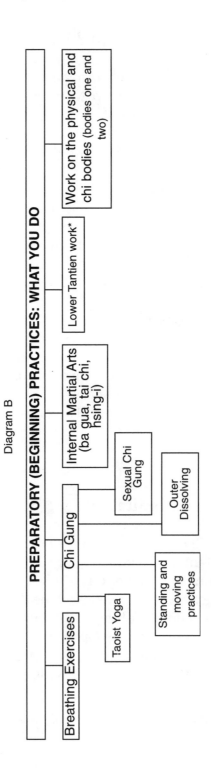

PREPARATORY (BEGINNING) PRACTICES: WHAT YOU DO

*There are three main tantiens (pronounced "dandiens"), or energy centers, in the human body. These are the places where chi collects and governs a person's energetic anatomy. The lower tantien, located just below the navel in the center of the body, is the energetic center primarily responsible for the health of the human body and the only center where all the energies that affect the physical body interact. The middle tantien has two locations: at the solar plexus and at the center of the chest near the heart (we will refer to this latter location as the middle tantien throughout the book). The first governs the functions of the middle internal organs; the second governs relationships with sentient beings. The upper tantien, located in the brain, controls human perceptual mechanisms and psychic functions.

Intermediate (Middle) Practices

The aim of the middle practices is to attain inner stillness and to become aware of Universal Consciousness. The benefits of the middle practices include gaining emotional harmony and releasing structural blockages in your emotions, including traumas and fixations.

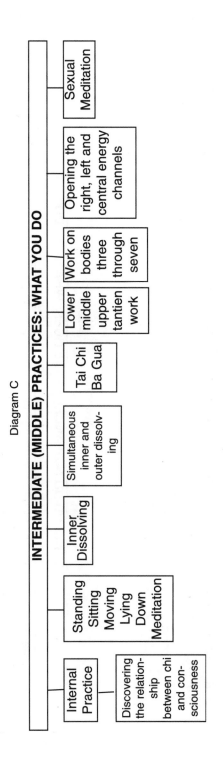

Diagram C

Concluding (Advanced) Practices

The aim of the advanced practices is to create the type of consciousness you wish to manifest until you decide to change it, that is, create your own vibratory frequency. The benefit sought is to become one with the Universal Consciousness (Tao).

Diagram D

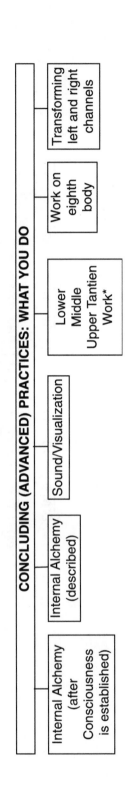

*See footnote on Diagram B, p. 34

stage. It will be useful to refer back to these diagrams as you read through the book.

Whatever you do, please do not attempt any intermediate or advanced practice before you can do all the preparatory work. The preparatory work is just that—it prepares your body to handle what comes after. The progression has valid reasons for being the way it is. It is recommended that you follow it.

You can begin practicing the preparatory exercises at once. Start with the breathing lesson in the Focus on Practice box on page 39. This is the first of twelve breathing lessons spaced throughout this book.

The 70 Percent Rule: The Foundation of All Taoist Water Method Practices

You are about to start Taoist internal breathing lessons. For all the lessons in this series about complete Taoist breathing, remember to take the limits of your concentration only to a maximum of 70 percent of your capacity (this is a general rule for all modes of practice). Inhale and exhale only 70 percent of what you could push yourself to do at your most extreme effort. This guideline allows you a comfort zone for your body, your central nervous system, and your ability to breathe and concentrate, so you can do the activity in a relaxed fashion that reduces, rather than increases, internal stress.

Beginning from an effortless position, you may, over time, gradually increase the duration of the in-breath and out-breath, along with the intensity with which the mind penetrates the internal sensations of the body and its energy. With this gradual progression, the action of breathing itself will induce relaxation and calmness in your body. With the 70 percent rule, it becomes *more relaxing*, over time, as you extend your breath from ten seconds to thirty seconds, to one minute, to two minutes--a shift that should bring major benefits to you over the course of your lifetime.

In all water method Taoist practices, the 70 percent rule permits you to become comfortable and relaxed when you do exert 100 percent of your unreserved, non-tension-bound effort on the activity at hand. As you get better and better and significantly extend your capacities with practice, if you stay with the 70 percent rule, you will be able to accomplish controlled breathing in a relaxed, comfortable, and effortless state of being.

Always apply the 70 percent rule to the practices suggested in this book. In fact, the 70 percent rule ideally should apply to every water method Taoist practice (see Question 7 in Appendix A).

Taoist Breathing Exercises

The big challenge in the preparatory phase of Taoist meditation is learning to concentrate on what you are doing for an extended time without becoming distracted. One of the best ways to achieve this ability is through breathing exercises. The Taoist breathing exercises form one of the building blocks of chi gung, the internal martial arts (ba gua, tai chi, and hsing-i), Taoist yoga, and Taoist meditation. These exercises are also used by chi therapists when applying their hands-on healing body/energy work. The exercises are immensely valuable for reducing stress and for building stamina, because the strength or weakness of the breath is a major factor in determining the mind's clarity and the body's health and vitality. In China they speak of controlling the "monkey mind," meaning a mind that jumps from place to place and has trouble getting to the center of an issue. Certainly, impatience has become a serious problem in our age of electronics, where ten seconds is considered a "long time."

The twelve breathing lessons presented throughout this book are designed to give you internal strength and to gradually enable your mind to settle and concentrate for long periods of time on whatever you choose. Moreover, this practice, done consistently, will awaken the energy of your lower tantien (the *hara* in Japanese, *ka* in Sufism), the fundamental energy center for all beginning Taoist practices of meditation, healing, or psychic development. When you are satisfied that you can do one lesson, go on to the next. Progress at your own pace.

The primary purpose of learning these breathing lessons is, then, to give you a technique to train your awareness so that you can use it to become conscious of the inside of your physical body and its energies. Remember to always

FOCUS ON PRACTICE
Taoist Internal Breathing, Lesson 1:
Feeling the Breath

 Stand or sit comfortably with eyes and mouth closed. Place the tip of your tongue on the roof of your mouth and gently rest it there. Relax all the muscles of your face. Let your mind become aware of your breath entering your nostrils as you inhale and exhale. Feel all the sensations (physical and nonphysical) to the end of the inside of your nostrils, including the movement of your nose hairs.

After you can feel the movement of breath inside your nose, continue following the sensation of your breath in stages. As you become aware of the breath itself, let your breath penetrate progressively down the center line of your body and feel everything along the way. First, to the bottom of your throat. Next, to your lungs, your solar plexus, your navel, and then your lower tantien, which is approximately one-third of the distance between your navel and genitals. Practice five to ten minutes or more, keeping in mind the 70 percent rule, so you progressively relax, avoiding strain to either your body, breath, or mind.

This is a general breathing process. In the lessons that follow, the breathing process will be described in greater detail.

breathe in and out through your nose unless some medical condition precludes it. In the beginning, perform the breathing lessons in a standing or sitting position and avoid drafty, cold, or damp places.

Who Are the Taoists?

In order to fully comprehend and appreciate the Taoist meditative practices, it is necessary to know something of the context in which these techniques originated.

Many Westerners are under the mistaken impression that large numbers of Chinese are Taoists. In China it is commonly held, however, that practicing Taoists are less than one percent of that country's population. Most Taoist practice in modern China is commingled with facets of Buddhism and folk religion. Be that as it may, a pure, distinct Taoist tradition does indeed exist, and the Buddhist and the Taoist ways of looking at the same phenomena are often somewhat different.

Taoists have never really pushed to gain adherents. More often than not in Chinese history they have actively discouraged membership or have gone underground. The last time the Taoists were really public and had patronage of the ruling class in China was during the Tang dynasty (618–907 A.D.). This period is considered by many historians to be China's most creative.

Whether exoteric or esoteric in nature, most religions, when given the opportunity, will try to build as large an empire as possible. They strive for cohesive influence over great numbers. Witness the giants—Christianity, Islam, Hinduism, Buddhism. The major branches of Taoism have never demonstrated any particular desire, using meditation or belief systems, to build theocratic empires.

The Taoist tradition has always been essentially what could be called mystical rather than organizational. Practitioners of this tradition have been primarily focused on exploring the quintessential spiritual nature of human beings, including people's relationship to their environment, their inner selves, and the universe. Taoists consider almost everything that happens in the external world (beliefs, events, opinions, hopes, fears) to be what they refer to as "red dust"—things come, stay for awhile, and go as the wind blows (see p. 105). The main Taoist work, the classic *I Ching* or *Book of Changes* attempts to comprehend change and changelessness from many different viewpoints. Through sixty-four systematically presented real-life situations called *hexagrams*, the *I Ching* teaches that everything in the world is in continual flux. Through meditation, a Taoist aims to discover that which never changes and is always present. Hexagrams, like the *trigrams* that combine to form them, are concerned with change and with the empty space in the midst of that which is changeless, the Tao.

Taoists in China have been a very strange group. Many have been talented, educated, and powerful, with some holding prestigious positions before they renounced the world. For example, Lao Tse, the author of the *Tao Te Ching*, was the head librarian of the imperial archives when only the elite could read. He was responsible for maintaining all the written knowledge in China at the time.

Chang San Feng, the Taoist immortal* who some believe was the founder of tai chi chuan, was a major magistrate before becoming a Taoist. Lu Tsu (also known as Lu Tung Pin), a major Taoist immortal whose followers are commonly considered to constitute the greatest group of fully realized Taoist sage/immortals, was also said to be a magistrate, a rank that is today more or less the equivalent of a senior government official.**

---

*A Taoist immortal is someone who, in Taoism, has actualized all eight energy bodies (see p. 50). An immortal's consciousness has merged with the Tao.

**The position of a magistrate in a feudal society carried with it much more overt control than that of a powerful official in a democracy. The Chinese magistrate, for example, had life-and-death power over people and could act purely on his whims and moods.

THE WAY OF LIU
My Teacher, the Master Liu Hung Chieh

 Liu was a short, thin man who possessed extraordinarily strong internal power and a subtlety of movement unique even among the foremost martial arts masters of Asia. His mind was penetrating and clear, encompassing an intelligence of high order. His ability to communicate the most mysterious aspects of Taoism without digression was the mark of a true genius, and the power of his mind was surpassed only by the internal balance and compassion of his heart. Through his studies and his arduous training, Liu eventually became one of those extremely rare individuals who ascended to be designated a living Taoist immortal. Liu's mastery of Taoism progressed in three distinct phases.

In his youth, Liu was a staunch Confucian, born into a wealthy landowning family of ten generations of Chinese doctors. During middle school, he was the last and youngest member to be initiated into the original ba gua martial arts school in Beijing.* There, during his teens and twenties, he learned the meditation approach of that school, techniques based on the *I Ching*. An avid and talented student of classical Chinese literature, Liu graduated from one of the universities from which the modern Beijing University was established. He taught at the university level for a short while before pursuing his other main loves of martial arts and meditation full-time. He was, however, never distant from his scholarly pursuits. After representing the ba gua school at China's first modern National Martial Arts Competition in 1928, he became head of instructors at the National Martial Arts Institute in Changsha, Henan Province, for three years.**

In middle age, after becoming an accomplished master of the internal martial arts of hsing-i and ba gua, he went to Hong Kong and lived in the home of Wu Jien Chuan, who along with his father cofounded the Wu style of tai chi.

*Ba gua chang is a complex Taoist martial art based on the *I Ching*.

**See B. K. Frantzis, *The Power of Internal Martial Arts* (Berkeley, Calif.: North Atlantic Books, 1998), pp. 241–247.

THE WAY OF LIU
My Teacher, the Master Liu Hung Chieh (continued)

There Liu learned Wu's tai chi thoroughly and became one of Wu's teaching assistants. Liu also attended a lecture by the head of the Tien Tai school of Buddhism in Beijing. He was so deeply impressed by the message of the dharma that he entered the master's monastery as a student. His progress there was so remarkable that after a brief few years he was formally declared enlightened in Mahayana Buddhism by Tan Hsiu Fa Shr, the head of the Tien Tai sect. Liu now turned toward the Tao. He traveled to the sacred mountains of Western China, where for ten years he devoted himself to intense study with a number of those meditation masters who head the esoteric branches of Taoism that extend back to antiquity through an unbroken line of lineage masters.

The third phase of Liu's life began in 1949 when he returned from the mountains to Beijing. He had intended to take his family to Taiwan or Hong Kong, but was prevented from doing so by political circumstances. Liu stayed in Beijing until his death on December 1, 1986. During those years, he was virtually an urban hermit within Beijing. He willingly took on the incredibly difficult task of living in Communist China while devoting himself solely to practicing Taoist inner alchemy and quietly performing his duties as the head of a Taoist sect.

FOCUS ON PRACTICE
Taoist Internal Breathing, Lesson 2

- Place the tip of your tongue on the roof (hard palate) of your mouth.

- Take a complete breath. A complete breath consists of a smooth inhale and exhale with no holding of the breath whatsoever after the end of either the inhale or the exhale.

- Gradually make your breath longer and longer. To the best of your ability, each breath should be quiet, soft, and relaxed. Practice for five or ten minutes.

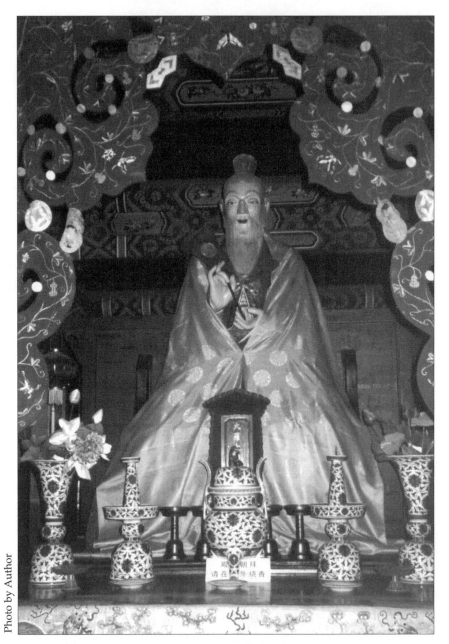

Statue of Daode Tianzun, a deified incarnation of Lao Tse, from the White Cloud Temple (Bai Yun Guan) in Beijing. This has been the most important Taoist temple in China since the Mongol invasions seven hundred years ago.

Taoism in Perspective

CHAPTER 2

Chuang Tzu Metamorphosis

Four men were talking and said
"Does someone know how to have
The Void for his head
Life for his spine and
Death for his tail?
This one shall be my friend."
Looking in each others' spirit
They nodded in agreement
Started laughing
And became friends

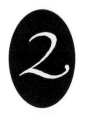

Taoism in Perspective

In general, Taoists have been self-motivated individuals who have sought to function from the drives of their own inner awareness rather than external circumstances. Prevailing societal beliefs have been irrelevant to them. Being independent spirits, they might or might not follow established social conventions. Historically, many were people who had gone into life, were generally successful, and reaped the rewards, but at a certain point said to themselves, "I don't know—all the power, all these rules! Is this what life in the universe is all about?"

Many got fed up with the world. It was not so much that these Taoists left the world, it was more as if the world left them. Feeling this, they lacked any concern about what conventional society considered to be important—they had come to recognize the limitations of external appearances. They didn't care if they uplifted people or upset them, and could not have cared less what people thought of them. They lost interest in physical image. Where in their pre-Taoist days they may have worn bejeweled robes of the finest silks, as Taoists they often went about in rags, completely content. As Taoists, their full focus was now directed toward comprehending the essence of being. For them, the prime question became, "What is all of this in here and out there?" These individuals were serious about studying the essential nature of their inner beings and the phenomenon of the universe, while at the same time not taking themselves seriously.

One of the goals of every Taoist is to understand the energy of any individual, object, event, or interaction. Gaining such understanding is the basic theme of the *I Ching*, the oldest central text of all schools of Taoism. Taoists believe that so many different energies manifest (that is, take on a recognizable form) in the universe that we cannot easily perceive that there is a central underlying energetic process (the Tao) that fuels all manifestation. Thus we become confused by appearances and lose touch with the core reality of the Tao. In Taoism, one way of eliminating that confusion is simply to accept that any given energy is what it is, regardless of what form or shape it has or what psychological impact it is producing at the moment. Thus Taoists will involve themselves in all manner of activities where they fully assume and emanate the energy of that activity, purely to experience it for what it is. For example, in the martial arts you might witness a Taoist who when meditating is quiet and gentle but when fighting exhibits a roughness that would make the fiercest warrior seem friendly. Yet the Taoist does not judge one state of being as "better" than the other. Each state has its natural and useful time and place—one can learn from both.

The energy of meditation or fighting or healing has a specific and distinct nature, as though it were a concrete thing. It is just what it is. To the Taoist, when you express the energy of a specific phenomenon, it simply means that you have manifested one specific energy that exists—you are not it, and it is not you, much in the same way as when changing a shirt, you are not the shirt. Rather, the shirt is only a "something" you use.

After lengthy and continuous meditative practice, the adept Taoist student gains the ability to shape energy and in the process learns how to accept any energy for what it is, not needing to make it other than what it intrinsically may be. Many people spend a good portion of their lives fighting the conditions around them, wanting energy to be different from what it is, wanting people to be other than what they are, wanting life to be different from what it is, wanting to twist some aspect of life's energy into something it is not. While certainly energies can be opposed and changed (as in the case of those energies that are destructive or evil), the capacity to recognize naturally occurring phenomena simply for what they are is one of the greatest challenges in life, one that most people do not take on.

Taoists of the Right and Left

As with most groups, Taoists have right and left contingents (or conservatives and liberals, if you prefer). The bulk of the Taoists, however, are in the center. They go about their meditation practices by themselves or in small, sometimes interconnected groups, meeting members of other groups for a variety of secular and spiritual purposes. Centrist Taoists lead normal lives. They go to school, have jobs, own businesses, and raise families.

Traditionally, the right-wing or conservative Taoists in China tended to isolate themselves in the mountains, where they struggled to attain spiritual clarity and balance (that is, connection with the universal Tao) primarily by using moving and seated meditation techniques. The right-wingers attempted to achieve wisdom and peace through a highly regulated, moderate, and often celibate lifestyle that was fairly quiet. In this way, they gradually disengaged from the distractions of worldly life. They often lived in small, secluded mountain communities, either alone or in groups of three to five. Lone hermits or small groups sometimes resided inside a cave or mountain hermitage, perhaps not emerging for fifty years. Less often, they banded together in monasteries, which were not nearly as big as the hugely populated monasteries one can find in the history of Buddhism and Christianity.

In stark contrast, the wandering left-wing Taoists were known for being outrageous in their lifestyles and sexual behavior. There was nothing a leftist Taoist would not do. Taoists of the left frequently scorned or ignored social conventions and expectations outright. But while they often repudiated many specific aspects and values of society, they (and this is an important point) adhered to awareness in all they did, avoided causing harm, and attempted to balance all they came in contact with.

Like the Taoists of the right, those of the left would do all of the sitting and moving practices but, unlike the rightists, would afterward try to bring the results of their meditation into their daily lives. They deliberately moved and refined their internal energies as they engaged in real-life activities, all with the goal of learning to transform themselves in life's swirling cauldron of unpredictability. Life's daily pleasures, sexual and otherwise, as well as disasters and turmoil, became the impetus for their meditation practice. Practitioners of the left used the situations and energies (both safe and dangerous) of real-life resources to transform their internal blockages into internal harmony.

If you walk the left-hand path of Taoism, you will meditate and then will find yourself deliberately entering into situations where you continually risk all of your most cherished images of your self. Detached, but with the goal of acutely sharpening awareness, Taoists of the left play quite actively with the world, indulging in sex, politics, business, and so on.

In China Taoists have a reputation for being reclusive. Yet the Taoists I met there were, on the whole, extremely open minded and happy at times to reveal their practices. In the past Taoists have tended to conceal who they were or what they were doing to avoid persecution. The tormenting of nonconformists is certainly nothing new. As it was in the Spanish Inquisition or in ancient Greece, where Socrates was forced to swallow hemlock for his independent thinking, so it was for the Taoists throughout much of Confucian Chinese history.

The Eight Bodies

Given their preoccupation with energy and its study, Taoists have identified in humans a system of distinct vibrational levels of energy that they call the "Eight Bodies." They believe that each person possesses eight different energy bodies.

FOCUS ON PRACTICE
Taoist Internal Breathing, Lesson 3

- Consciously count each of your breaths, first for 2 breaths, then 3, then 4, then 5, then 6, then 7, then 8, then 9, and finally 10 breaths, without losing count or spacing out.

- Begin with one set of 10 breaths. Progressively build to 2 sets of 10 breaths, then 3, then 4, then 5 sets of 10 breaths until, without getting distracted, you feel each inhale and exhale. Be sharply aware of your count.

- In the beginning, you can use your fingers or beads to keep count, but eventually you will want to keep track without any external support, thereby strengthening your mind's awareness and continuity.

- Do your best to breathe and count in a relaxed manner, without tensing up. While counting, do not project into the future. Concentrate on the breath going through your body at the instant it is doing so.

The first is your *physical body*, which is the most dense of the human energy bodies. The succeeding bodies consist of progressively more subtle energies that vibrate at higher and higher frequencies. Beginning with the physical body, each successive body not only occupies the same space as the previous one but also extends farther outward and therefore is larger than the one before. Your consciousness of your physical body ideally should begin inside your bone marrow and extend outward to your skin.

The second is your *chi body*, which coexists within the same space as your physical body and, along an undifferentiated continuum without gaps, extends outward, away from all the surfaces of your skin, anywhere from a few inches in an ill person to two or more feet in an energetically vibrant person. (In Western esoterica and in both volumes of this book, this energetic layer just beyond the skin is also inter-changeably known as the *etheric body* or *aura*..) It vibrates at a slightly higher frequency than the physical body and is significantly less dense. The chi body fuels the physical body. It is the body with which acupuncture and chi gung exercises work. Such chi is found only in the living; it does not reside in a corpse.

The third body is the even more subtle, even higher-frequency *emotional body*, which the Taoists believe extends far outside of the physical body deep into space, as do the subsequent bodies, each one progressively more subtle and expansive. In Taoist meditation one works this body to liber-ate the emotions by removing emotional energy blocks that the Chinese call "ghosts" or "demons." Through such prac-tices you rid yourself of the negative emotional residues from childhood and later experiences and break the restraints that come from how you were conditioned to live by your parents, teachers, and role models. Such liberation enables you to take full responsibility for your own emotions. Sitting meditation practices are crucial in this process.

The refinement of the fourth or *mental body* enhances the mind's ability to discriminate between what Taoists call "the real and the false." Necessary to this is the opening of the brain energy centers of the upper tantien. It is from clarity at this level of energy that great intellectual accomplishments and the capacity for clear, instantaneous decisions are derived. If the third or emotional body is not fully devel-oped, however, this fourth body will not function fully. Your emotions can and do easily fog and even override your mental energies. Each higher energetic body has a more powerful ability to influence the lower bodies than vice versa. Nonetheless, without the support of the preceding lower body, the next higher will be unable to manifest its full power.

Development of the fifth, or *psychic energy body*, more subtle yet, allows us to find our hidden internal capacities. Primary among these are perception of the unseen or "spirit" world, the awareness of energy within solid matter, and intuition about events of which one has no direct knowledge, such as information gained through clairvoyance or clairaudience. When you are able to use the energies on this level, you become experientially aware of the invisible world described in the shamanic traditions. The Taoists view these as natural human abilities that have become blocked in most people (sometimes for their own safety and the safety of others). Once the energy of the emotional and mental bodies has developed sufficiently and your power to discriminate between reality, fantasy, and self-delusion has also developed, there is little or no danger involved in being open to the unseen world. If, on the other hand, your lower bodies are not adequately prepared, opening the psychic body can be mentally or emotionally destabilizing.

The *causal body*, the sixth, is the body related to time and space. At this subtle vibratory frequency exist the energies that cause events to manifest in the physical world and in time and space (from huge events, such as the creation and demise of galaxies, to smaller events, such as the precise time, place, and circumstances of human birth and death). It is this level of energy to which you connect when you throw the *I Ching* coins or stalks for purposes of divination. A reasonably stable center of stillness within your innermost being is absolutely essential to work at this level of energy. Here you use a balance of your moving and sitting meditation practices to ensure that your physical body does not get "blown out" by the enormous amount of energy passing through it. During work at this level, not only will the energy of your sense of "I" crystallize and become apparent, but you will also see the energies responsible for the laws of cause and effect. The Taoists say that someone who masters this level of practice can achieve physical immortality, but not necessarily spiritual immortality, that is, complete, not partial, union with the Tao.

It is the cultivation of the seventh body, or *body of individuality*, that entails the actual birth of the full spiritual being. Initially, all of us are what the *I Ching* calls the "inferior person" ("man" has been the general translation used in the West, but the original language uses the word "person"), meaning that, within us, the different energy bodies are separate, uncoordinated, and unclear. The word *inferior* does not contain a judgmental quality but refers rather to the degree of a person's overall spiritual development. When you become one with the seventh body, the energy of your ego first reaches its full potential and then completely dissolves. At this point, the separate energies of your first seven bodies become unified and you change into what in the West is commonly referred to as someone who is illuminated, enlightened, or self-realized. That is, you are freed from your lower nature and exist as the "superior person" of the *I Ching*. The mind of the superior person listens to and follows the mind of the Tao, but the superior person is not one with the Tao. Rather, such individuals become one with themselves and one with the earth. This state is the culmination of the intermediate stage of Taoist meditation which the Taoists call *The Great Stillness*, and the Chinese Buddhists commonly designate as "enlightenment." Some Buddhist sects and some Hindus believe that to go further and join with the whole of the universe a person must die and leave the body. The Taoists, in contrast, believe such joining can be done while one is still in one's body.

The eighth energy body is called the *body of the Tao*. This energetic level entails the joining of the human consciousness to the whole of the universe. In other words, to fully realize the eighth body is to achieve utter and complete unity with the Tao. This is the ultimate point of Taoist energy work. Those who arrive at this state are said to be "guardians of the worlds." They are also the only ones who traditionally have earned the right to be called Taoist immortals. The Taoists believe that you are unconsciously already enlightened. When the light that is inside you shines, it can sometimes be frightening. The Taoists note reassuringly that when you literally look at the whole of eternity, there is nothing unusual about being overwhelmed. Just relax. The Tao exists, and sooner or later, through your meditative practice, you will become aware of it.

FOCUS ON A SPECIAL TOPIC
The Sixteen-Part Nei Gung System

 The energetic work of Taoist meditation is based on a sixteen-part *nei gung* system.* This system of energetic exercise is most likely the root from which all the other chi gung systems in China have arisen.** It is also the root of the essential Chi work of the internal martial arts of ba gua, tai chi, and hsing-i, of Chi therapy and bodywork, and of Taoist meditation. Just as a circle continues around only to return to its origin, the sequence of learning the sixteen components is flexible. Where you start is determined by your goal—for example, increasing capability for high performance, improving personal health, learning martial arts, learning to heal others, or advancing in meditation.

The sixteen basic components of Taoist nei gung include:

1. Breathing methods, from the simple to the more complex.
2. Feeling, moving, transforming, and transmuting internal energies along the descending, ascending, and connecting energy channels of the body.
3. Precise body alignments to prevent the flow of chi from being blocked or dissipated; practicing these principles brings exceptionally effective biomechanical alignments.
4. Dissolving blockages of the physical, emotional, and spiritual aspects of ourselves.
5. Moving energy through the main and secondary meridian channels of the body, including the energy gates.

*My instructors and I teach these energetic practices in a systematic six-part chi gung program. These particular chi gung practices have been passed down unchanged for thousands of years. They have withstood the test of time, and continue to work extremely well. See p. 206 for more information.

**The other main chi gung systems in China are Buddhist, martial arts, medical, and Confucian. Despite a common sharing of techniques among them, there are also differing specializations, goals, and philosophical tenets from one to the next. For more information concerning the relationship between the sixteen-part nei gung system and the martial arts, see Frantzis, *The Power of Internal Martial Arts*, pp. 62–76.

FOCUS ON A SPECIAL TOPIC
The Sixteen-Part Nei Gung System (continued)

6. Bending and stretching the body from the inside out and from the outside in, along the direction of the yin and yang acupuncture meridian lines.
7. Opening and closing all parts of the physical body (joints, muscles, soft tissues, internal organs, glands, blood vessels, cerebrospinal system, and brain), as well as all aspects of the body's subtle energy anatomy.
8. Manipulating the energy of the external aura outside the body.
9. Making circles and spirals of energy inside the body, controlling the spiraling energy currents of the body, and moving energy to any part of the body at will, especially to the glands, brain, and internal organs.
10. Absorbing energy into, and projecting energy away from, any part of the body.
11. Controlling all the energies of the spine.
12. Gaining control of the left and right energy channels of the body.
13. Gaining control of the central energy channel of the body.
14. Learning to develop the capabilities and all the uses of the body's lower tantien.
15. Learning to develop the capabilities and all the uses of the body's upper and middle tantiens.
16. Connecting every part of the physical and other energetic bodies into one unified energy.

The Three Treasures and Emptiness

The workings of the eight bodies of a human are also looked at as the transformational interplay between the three treasures of body, energy, and spirit and the creation of the emptiness that eventually leads an individual to the Tao. Everything in the whole of creation, including the energy of the body, is perceived by Taoists in terms of the qualities of raw and refined energy. Raw energy—the first treasure, body—is considered to be a commingling of three different kinds of energy: (1) that which comprises the physical body (bone, blood, tissues, organs, etc.); (2) that which fuels the physical body, the chi that moves through acupuncture meridians and makes everything in the body work; and (3) that which is expressed in gross, instinctual emotional energy (like that of an enraged or cringing animal, for example).

Refined energy—the second treasure, Chi—is considered to be a commingling of two different kinds of energy: (1) that which runs your lower mental body—that is, the power that gives you the strength to think, at least at a concrete level, and (2) that which allows you to perceive your higher emotions (those that are not strictly concerned with self, such as compassion and love). In Taoist meditative practices, the raw energy of the physical body (*jing*) is refined and converted to chi. When this chi stabilizes (that is to say, when it is no longer random and confused), it becomes refined into Chi, and this Chi, as it becomes refined, will begin to produce spirit.*

When you begin to experience spirit—the third treasure—you move into the depths of your awareness and essence—you begin to realize at the very core of your being that which is not bound by time and space. At the level of spirit, you begin to become spiritually alive, connected with

---

*In Taoism the word *spirit* has different meanings depending on the context. In Chinese medicine it refers to the vibrancy of an individual's entire physical and mental condition. That is not what is meant here. The word spirit in Taoist meditation refers specifically to the fifth and sixth energetic levels—the psychic and causal, respectively.

The distinction between the terms *Chi* and *spirit* in the Taoist meditation traditions sometimes causes confusion. Although energetically Chi and spirit are not the same, in those cases where they become commingled and mutually affect each other, the word *Chi* is used to refer to both. Whether Chi or spirit plays the more important role in the sentence, paragraph, or entire discussion is determined by context. That context may be overt or subtle, with many hidden underlying assumptions concerning energy flows of which a nonpractitioner may not be aware.

FOCUS ON A SPECIAL TOPIC
Jing (Body), Chi (Energy), Shen (Spirit)

 In Chinese, the core progression of Taoist meditation practice is expressed as:

jing	*Chi*	*shen*	*wu*	*Tao*
body	energy	spirit	emptiness	path

The evolution of Taoist practice as represented by this progression is:

jing, or physical body (energy, or sperm),* begets
Chi, or energy, which begets
shen, or spirit, which begets
wu, or emptiness, which begets
the *Tao*, which is the essential, unchanging root
of the universe.

The concept of "body" includes everything in us that is corporeal: our gross anatomy, the physical body (the first of the eight bodies); the chi that makes the physical body work, that makes it live (the second of the eight bodies); and the energy expressed by the lower emotions (the primal animal emotions, such as anger and fear).

The concept of Chi in this system includes the third and fourth energetic bodies, encompassing the lower mental functions (that is, the energy that permits thought on a concrete level, such as "that is a tree" or "open the door") and the higher mental functions (the capacity for abstract and analytical thought and the ability to have direct perception of the nature of things). The concept of Chi also includes sensitivity to the higher emotions (those more abstract emotions that tend to include feelings over and above the self, such as kindness or love).

Spirit, or soul, begins to be formed at the energy levels of the psychic and causal bodies (the fifth and sixth energetic bodies). It grows until it touches emptiness in the causal body and then enters emptiness for additional transformation, until emptiness stabilizes in the body of individuality. You must have first reached the stage of Great Stillness (as described in this volume's final chapter) for this progression of the spirit from emptiness to the Tao to occur.

*The word *jing* literally translates as "sperm," but the concept here is that it is the sperm (or egg) that creates a physical body, so *jing* is the energy of the physical body.

yourself, others, and the environment in a profound, unified way—a genuine spiritual process has begun.

With additional practice you will start experiencing emptiness. Everything will seem to be without content. Ordinarily, we experience both external and internal objects in the world as having shape, size, and some kind of content. Everything has an inherent identification or meaning that the mind can grasp. As emptiness is accessed through meditation, however, your spirit starts increasingly to transform the energies of your perceptions of solid objects and stored mental images. Even though another person or a house or tree or airplane is still present (that is, exists for you), they are experienced as having no substance. They are literally nothing (emptiness). As you start perceiving every tangible thing as nothing, you discover that nothingness simultaneously becomes full of Universal Consciousness, which is potentially able to become anything. There is no difference between everything being nothing and nothing being everything. Your ongoing awareness spans the tremendous spiritual dichotomy between emptiness and fullness/form. You keep playing with this paradox, back and forth. It usually takes a lot of meditative practice to get to this point. But when there, once in a while you spontaneously catch a glimpse of the unchanging source of emptiness and fullness that cannot be expressed verbally. There quite literally are no words to describe what you become aware of. It is just what it is. It is known by many names in many traditions; the Chinese call it the Tao.

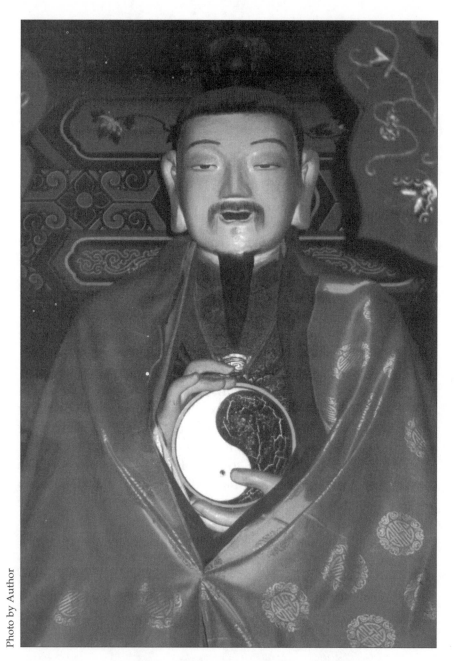

Statue from the White Cloud Temple in Beijing, China of Lingbao Tianzun, one of the Three Pure Gods. Each of the gods embodies a quality of the deified Lao Tse.

Water and Fire:
Two Methods of Meditation

CHAPTER
3

Lao Tse Tao Te Ching, Verses 53 and 81

The Great Tao is not hard
Yet people choose side doors that deviate from the true
Pay attention when things become unbalanced
Center yourself within the Tao

The Tao sustains and furthers all
by not straining or using force

Water and Fire:
Two Methods of Meditation

There are two main methods of Chinese Taoist meditation: the fire and water approaches. The fire method emphasizes force and pushing forward. It has the characteristics of flame, ever leaping forward to consume more fuel. The water method, on the other hand, believes in effort without force, in relaxation, in letting go. It displays the characteristics of water: softness and flow.

The Water Method: An Orientation

The original water school of Taoism came into flower during Lao Tse's time, around twenty-five hundred years ago. Unlike the Neo-Taoist fire tradition, the original water school Taoists had no great drive toward physical immortality, a major focus of Neo-Taoism.* While the water method is known for not forcing things, for literally letting things occur in their own time, it is far from passive. Adherents of the water method prepare in every possible way so that when circumstances are ripe for the successful completion of their practice, they are fully open and available to the moment.

---

*Neo-Taoism is a major branch of Taoism that came into being in third-century China. It combines Taoist metaphysics with Confucian social and political philosophy. A review of Neo-Taoism appears in *A Sourcebook in Chinese Philosophy*, translated and compiled by Wing-Tsit Chan (Princeton, N.J.: Princeton University Press, 1963).

The Taoist water meditation tradition, deeply rooted in the *I Ching*, had a thousand-year history behind it before Lao Tse appeared. Lao Tse did not originate the water method tradition or its basic principles by any means, but he was the first one to record them in writing. He wrote the *Tao Te Ching* on his journey out of the country, trying to get away from worldly life. One of his students, a border guard, refused Lao Tse passage, demanding that he leave behind some principles in writing before he left the country and went into seclusion.

The water method is a practical way to release blockages in the whole mind/body so one can fully transform and ultimately experience conscious harmony with the Tao, right down to one's bone marrow. Then one naturally acts according to the principles of the *Tao Te Ching*.*

The water practices are based on a philosophical perspective that is relevant to everyday life: *Whatever you do must feel comfortable.* You learn to exert full effort without strained force. In order to do that, you must refine a certain edge in the mind. To employ all of your effort and yet not use force, not contravene the actual limits of the body, the mind, and the spirit, is the gentle way of Lao Tse.

Taoist water method practices are divided into preparatory, intermediate, and advanced stages (see Diagrams B–D in Chapter 1). Once again, it is important to complete the training at one stage before progressing to the next.

The Dissolving Practice: Initial Descriptions

The core and most essential practice of the water method of meditation is to "dissolve" or release bound

---

*Many of the phrases of the *Tao Te Ching* are what might be called philosophical sound bites: one-line explanations that are simplified versions of complete and complicated practices in Taoism. For example, the phrase "the wise man breathes from his heels" refers to the whole progressive Taoist nei gung breathing and energy channel practices (see Chapter 2). These culminate in a person's directly taking in the energy of the earth through the etheric body into the feet and from there into all the body's energy channels.

energy in your body in order to make you free to merge with the Tao and be capable of perceiving it.

Taoists believe that since you inhabit this planet and are a physical being, you need to deal completely with the fact of your physicality—namely, your ability to feel and be fully conscious of whatever sensations are inside your body. Thus, you start water method meditation in Taoism by training your mind to focus attention fully on the sensations of energy in your body and your conscious awareness. The preparatory or beginning practices prepare you for entry into this area. The intermediate practice of dissolving immerses you directly in it.

When you start feeling deeply inside yourself, you often find places where your energies have become frozen; in some way, your physical body, chi, emotions, and so on, have congealed, closing down the channels and points through which energy flows in your body. All energy inside a human being, if it is free (that is, unlocked) is like a flowing river. Because of innumerable conditions and circumstances, however, we commonly do not retain the free-flowing energies that are ours at birth. The condensed or blocked energies assume an actual form or shape that is recognizable. Instead of an energy flowing freely, it becomes like water gathering in front of a dike or stagnating in a putrid pond. These condensed energetic shapes block the normal flow of Chi in your various energetic bodies, and such blockage can then cause you to become ill, dysfunctional, or diminished in some way. That is why the practice of chi gung (or energy work) almost invariably begins with techniques to dissolve blocked energy and move it outside the body.

Two Kinds of Dissolving

There are essentially two approaches for using your mind or awareness to release blocked energies in your body: the chi gung outer dissolving process, which may be done with the preparatory and intermediate practices, and the inner dissolving process of Taoist meditation, which normally begins only with the intermediate practices. The preparatory dissolving techniques may be done either standing or sitting, as described in greater detail in Chapter 5.

The objective of dissolving is to release any energy that has congealed into a specific shape—to make such energy become neutral and without boundaries. What is presented here is a brief introductory description of the two dissolving processes.* Both of these dissolving methods can be done by allowing your awareness to scan your body from top to bottom (downward), from bottom to top (upward), or in any number of directions. *This book deals specifically with the downward direction.* Learning to allow energy to flow downward first is a necessary safety precaution that prepares you to handle upward and other directional flows without injuring your central nervous system.

The Outer Dissolving Chi Gung Practice: The Transformation of Ice to Water to Gas

To dissolve outward, you use your mind to scan your body *downward* from head to toe, until you locate a place in your body where your energy is blocked or frozen, identified by a sensation of strength, tension, discomfort, or contraction. As your awareness becomes more sensitive, you can begin to feel or experience the outer contours of this frozen energy space. You should always stay alert for the slightly more subtle energy that exists behind the energy that is obviously felt (i.e., the layer beyond whichever you are currently dissolving.) Your awareness begins to enter into the obvious solid mass, causing the frozen energy to begin to soften, until you reach the center of the blockage. This is the transformation of ice to water. (If you put an ice cube in a pan and heat it on the stove, you will observe that the outside of the ice

---

*The second volume of this series, *The Great Stillness*, includes further instructions for both inner and outer dissolving, as well as practices to be done while lying down, moving, and during sexual activity.

cube melts first, with the melting progressing slowly toward the center of the cube.)

As the frozen energy in your body becomes soft or flowing (like the water in the pan), you keep your attention on that place and your awareness continues to cause that energy space to expand until there is a sense of the trapped energy expanding out beyond your skin, perhaps as much as a foot or two outside the surface. This is the transformation of water to gas. Like the water in the pan, which will not turn to gas until the ice cube is entirely liquefied, the dissolving of an energy block moves in stages.

To get a sense of this process, clench your fist as tight as you can, causing your energy to contract, until your knuckles turn white. Then feel your hand and expand your contracted energy until you completely relax your fist (ice to water). Then continue to focus your awareness on your closed hand until it feels discorporeal, empty of all solidity, with a completely amorphous quality which means your energy expands out of your hand into the air (water to gas).

This dissolving technique must be accomplished by feeling it, not only by picturing it in your mind's eye. Many people are extremely visual, and today visualization techniques are very common. The outer dissolving process, however, is not a visual experience at all; it is a *felt sensation*, in the same way you feel an ice cube or a candle on your hand.

The Inner Dissolving Taoist Meditation Practice: The Transformation of Ice to Water to Space

Chi gung's prime concern is developing physical health and strength. To achieve this goal it uses the outer dissolving technique to release trapped energy *externally* away from the body and into "outer space." Taoist meditation, in contrast, is primarily concerned with uncovering Universal Consciousness itself. Thus, the initial inner dissolving practices use the energy trapped within blockages as a fuel for moving yourself into unbound "inner space," ultimately imploding dissolved energy to the internal core of your being (that is, Consciousness itself). A phrase used in China for thousands of years to describe this process conveys the idea of "ice to water to inner space." The inner dissolving process is extremely helpful for resolving the temporary and long-term emotional, mental, and psychic stresses that can take much of the joy out of life. Through this process, the defined clump of frozen energy that was totally immovable becomes relaxed, amorphous, and flowing. Unbound energy can now go about its natural function, part of which is healing whatever ailment the original blockage caused. You then can move your mind deeper and deeper inside your energy field and consciousness, dissolving through layer after layer, until you trace each energy block back to its source. Eventually, the blockages will vanish, never to return, and you are freed from the prison of your energy blockages and can become one with the Tao.

FOCUS ON PRACTICE
Taoist Internal Breathing, Lesson 4

- Be very aware of—that is, *feel*—every sensation of each inhale and exhale.
- Feel the movement of the breath as it moves your nose hairs. How does each bit of breath make the inside of your nostrils feel?
- Follow and feel the connection of each micromovement of breath to your conscious awareness.
- Gradually build to 1 set of 10 breaths, staying acutely aware of how your mind follows each breath.
- Increase to 2 sets of 10 breaths, then 3, then 4, then 5 sets of 10 breaths, all the while concentrating on your conscious awareness.

The Fire Method: An Orientation

Contrasting to the water method are numerous fire traditions, one of which is the Neo-Taoist. Unaware that multiple traditions even exist, most Westerners are surprised to learn how much the traditions differ while simultaneously having many techniques in common. The techniques of the water and fire approaches, moreover, derive from divergent philosophical points of view. This situation has been the source of much confusion about the nature of Taoist practices, both in China and the West.*

Since the end of the Tang dynasty (618–907 A.D.), the fire traditions have been strongly influenced by Buddhist traditions, especially Tibetan tantric Buddhism. This Tibetan influence should not be surprising as, geographically, Tibet is as near to China's Sichuan province as Canada is to New York or Germany is to Switzerland.

The Neo-Taoists of the fire way are true believers in the idea that, in matters of spiritual attainment, the end justifies the means. Their methods are known for their willingness to emphasize force. They forcefully hold the breath, forcefully retain semen, and forcefully push past physical pain and mental and psychic discomfort to successfully complete a practice. They believe in "pushing forward" until they get to where they want to go. This point of view, to a certain degree, shows Buddhist influence. Why? Because in the fire school of Taoism any ascetic or self-inflicted pain is condoned or advocated if it allows one to become enlightened and "break the wheel of reincarnation" (Buddhist language) or create the "body of light" (both Buddhist tantric and Taoist fire school language). The basic belief here is that it doesn't matter what you do to yourself, because if in the end you become enlightened, anything you did was fine,

*Additional uncertainties arise around Taoism in America, where one finds a mixed bag of Taoist elements, including tai chi chuan, feng shui, and Chinese medicine. This book concentrates on the water method of Taoist meditation. The primary art of Taoist meditation, in each of its approaches, is something quite different from the Taoist martial and medical arts (see Diagram A in Chapter 1).

short of immoral or evil actions. There is a tremendous emphasis on pushing the limits in finding ways to rev up every energetic capacity of a human being. The Taoists of the water school hold a different point of view. They believe in effort without force, and that means and ends should essentially be the same.

One can clearly see fire aspects in the Buddhist traditions wherein Zen monks will sit in meditation indefinitely. Many of the enlightened in Zen have damaged their bodies considerably with their practices on the road to enlightenment. Actually, the Buddha himself did so during his years of asceticism, mortifying his body until he was virtually skin and bones. After his enlightenment, the Buddha preached against extreme practices. But many fire practitioners fixate on what the Buddha did in his early days rather than on his words *after wisdom had dawned.*

Fire melts metal—the metal of ego. Every fire tradition in the world is driven by the idea of conquest: "If there is an enemy, we will overcome it; if there is a wall, it will be gone through; if there is an ego, it will be slain; if there is a mountain, it must be climbed over, knocked down, picked up and dragged away." One has a constant sense, with followers of the fire method, that they absolutely must emerge a victor.

Another significant influence on the Neo-Taoist branch is the tradition of what they call in China *chi chi guai guai,* or "making strange things happen"—in short, magic. Advanced fire method meditators are said to be able to manipulate the energy for whatever reasons they have in mind. This accounts for the Neo-Taoists' noted obsession with developing certain energy channels for purposes of manifesting power, seen in desires such as, "I want to live to be a thousand years old" or "I want to be able to fly" or "I want to be able to leap over tall buildings with a single bound." It all boils down to, "I want the power to have this, and this, and make this and that happen, according to my will."

THE WAY OF LIU
Addiction to Psychic Power: The Traps

 In Taoist meditation, the initial object is to develop as much energy as possible, but not for the purpose of obtaining power. A desire for psychic (or paranormal) power is what in the early stages of meditation usually traps individuals—they become energy junkies. My teacher Liu put it very well. He said you would be better off with a vicious, self-destructive heroin or opium habit because then you would only need the opium; as soon as one life is over, the drug addiction is finished. But if you get addicted to psychic energy, the desire for that energy will endure for countless rebirths. Such addiction will not be something that you will be able to drop with the life that initiated the habit—it goes with you.

In Taoist practices, a tremendous amount of energy has to be developed inside the body in order for that energy to be converted to spirit. As your spirit fills, it is important that you start to realize the facts about the directions life can take, because when your spirit increases, you naturally gain what is known in the West as "personal power."

Through Taoist meditation, you can gather tremendous power, which is often not obvious to others.* If you stay focused on this power, then your spirit will never convert to emptiness (see Chapter 2). Being stuck on the power is considered "the big trap." As a matter of fact, virtually every esoteric tradition in the world holds that "the big trap" is to crave power. The character of the practitioner *must be developed* so he or she can willingly struggle with this problem and move beyond this trap.

Even upon reaching the advanced age of eighty, many human beings still live out the neuroses of their childhood.

---

*This refers to such psychic powers as (a) having one's energy flow into other people, animals, or power objects, a technique commonly developed in various spiritual and shamanistic traditions; (b) nonverbally influencing other people's minds, both at a distance and close up; (c) mentally dominating humans and animals; (d) having others crave you or be attracted to you, from a distance, with or without physical contact; (e) telekinesis and clairvoyance; (f) nonphysical energetic transmissions; and (g) controlling even small things, such as willing parking spaces to be available or having a needed taxi appear in the most unlikely circumstances.

THE WAY OF LIU
Addiction to Psychic Power: The Traps (continued)

They still relive things that occurred to them when they
were children or young adults. They never go beyond the
basic programmed conditioning wired inside them from
youth.

During the first level of Taoist water method meditation,
people spend a long time learning to become what Taoists
call "mature human beings," meaning individuals who can
assume responsibility for themselves, who do not avoid
consequences by ascribing their own motivations to others.
Possessing maturity is absolutely necessary before going
further. If you lack maturity when you start moving into the
world of spirit, you can become power mad and remain
hooked on power. In order to become free, you must throw
away whatever power and its benefits you have previously
accumulated.

The ego of people who acquire psychic power before
they are mature enough to handle it often inflates beyond
belief. An immature person who accumulates large amounts
of spiritual energy quickly and a youth who suddenly
becomes a fabulously rich rock star can experience similar
negative ego tendencies. Such people frequently abuse their
good fortune because they do not know how to produc-
tively channel the newly acquired energy, be it spiritual
power or money. The rock star frivolously spends millions
on drugs and childish whims, the spiritualist squanders
psychic energy on simple-minded gratification or domina-
tion games. The youth could, but does not, invest the cash;
the spiritualist could, but does not, heighten spiritual awareness to compassionately help fellow beings. Both have the
capacity to temporarily get what they want, without consid-
ering the effort that has brought them to this moment. They
forget that they can fall just as far as they have risen.

Adults have to pay the price for their actions, whereas
children are often forgiven on grounds of immaturity. In the
spiritual world, if you obtain power before you have
worked out the dark sides of your immature ego, trouble
can come your way. You may temporarily get away with all
sorts of nonsense, as many gurus do, but when you fall, you
become less than what you were before all your years of
practice. Maybe you "repent" or "wise up" and practice
again, until you reacquire your spiritual power and clarity.
But if the deepest underlying roots of your spiritual

THE WAY OF LIU
Addiction to Psychic Power: The Traps (continued)

immaturity are not dissolved and cleared, you can easily find yourself in an continuous spiritual cycle of boom and bust that can be avoided. The guideline is this: Emotional maturity is the absolutely necessary foundation upon which spiritual power must be built.

The Neo-Taoists' fascination with fire, force, opening channels, and having powerful awareness of what they can do with the energy they are producing often leads to a spiritual dead end. It rarely makes one spiritually free.*

*I draw this conclusion from a youth spent intensely experiencing the fire methods, as well as witnessing great numbers of people who have taken the fire method route.

The Fire and Water Methods Compared

The water method of Taoist meditation described in this book is in direct contrast to the fire methods of many traditions, Taoist and otherwise. For example, fire approaches include the extremely physical and emotive Hindu tantric and kundalini yoga traditions, with "kriyas" where people spontaneously shout, speak in tongues, do spontaneous yoga postures, curl into fetal positions, weep, yell, and growl like animals. Fire approaches include the Western psychological cathartic methods, such as encounter therapy, psychodrama with encouraged and guided screaming, hitting pillows, and releasing the full range of human emotions in highly dramatic ways. In the fire methods, there is always a tendency to keep pushing your energy outward (in fire language, releasing the fire in the cauldron of the lower tantien), releasing violent emotions explosively, or visualizing them as radiating light. All of these practices

FOCUS ON PRACTICE
Taoist Internal Breathing, Lesson 5:
Breathing Techniques to Increase
Conscious Awareness

- Extend your conscious awareness of each micro-inch of breath from your nostrils down to the base of your throat.
- Feel the front, sides, and back of your throat.
- Begin with 2 breaths, rest, then take 2 breaths again, and repeat until you can do 2 breaths successfully, *without breaking your awareness*. Now do 4 breaths, etc., until you can do 1 set of 10 breaths completely, with continuous awareness and no gross tension.
- Now work on 1 set of 10, having each breath relax every muscle and nerve in your body.
- Next work on relaxing the mental tension of your mind's conscious awareness on each breath. Keep at it until your attention can remain focused in a relaxed, comfortable manner.
- Gradually increase your breath work from 1 set of 10 breaths to 2, 3, 4, then 5 sets of 10.

have the potential to greatly irritate the central nervous system.

The water method Taoists say that the more energy is blocked, the more it should not be forced open. The more dense the anger and dysfunction, the greater the potential negative psychological repercussions if these suppressions are released too suddenly or explosively. Such negative repercussions include a destabilized central nervous system that makes it difficult for an individual to cope with the ordinary stress of life.

Different Interpretations of the Same Techniques

In their practices, both fire and water methods use many of the same techniques. Yet the specifics of how any technique may be used (such as where it occurs in a learning sequence), as well as the stated goals of the practice (that is, its value or meaning), may differ. For instance, a simple tai chi or martial art move may be performed in various ways depending on the style applied—small and condensed, expansive and large, or somewhere in the middle. Or consider meditation practiced to create inner stillness—fire schools will emphasize destroying, controlling, and otherwise transforming your negatively impacting internal energies right from the beginning, whereas water schools will emphasize dissolving, neutralizing, and releasing such energies first, and transforming them later.*

Both Fire and Water Methods Do Essentially the Same Channel Work but in Different Fashions

Both schools agree that the downward current of energy in the body must, for safety's sake, be stabilized before the upward current is activated. But the agreement on the use of energy ends there. Generally, fire method practitioners want to activate energy, make it move. Flame seeks any opportunity to jump and consume the next available fuel source; otherwise, it fades. Water, on the other hand, will move along the path of least resistance, but it is also content to stay motionless. Both types of energy have potential for

---

*The water school holds that there is a weak link in doing a transformation without first neutralizing the energy. Without such neutralization you may not release the secondary or underlying energies when you release the primary energy you are working on. The danger is that the secondary charges remain attached and will manifest in a different form in the newly transformed energy. For example, an unconscious, overtly aggressive, angry person can become (1) an unconscious, passive aggressive person; or (2) a person who is trying to be compassionate, yet is unconscious and oblivious to the negative effects of his or her actions, falsely believing them to be positive.

great power. A tidal wave is no less powerful than a volcano; a flood no less powerful than a forest fire.

The fire methods strongly emphasize using the mind both to create heat in the lower tantien and to deliberately control and move the Chi through the body's channels and points. The method entails keeping your intent on any blocked point in any given energy channel until you can push through it with your mind, thereby allowing Chi to move freely through the channel. In the water methods, the mind is used to apply the dissolving technique to naturally release any bound Chi in the body, without force, and without attempting to move forward until both body and mind are ready. The theory is that the Chi will move of its own accord into the appropriate channels with a minimum of prodding from the mind, just as water will seek its own level if left alone.

The fire method demands that the body listen to the commands of the mind; the water method seeks to allow the body to be able to hear the mind's commands. Both require actions to be natural. However, the fire school sometimes views the concept of "natural" from the reference point of not being satisfied with less than what the body/mind will be like after it is transformed. The water school, on the other hand, looks at what is comfortable and natural for you at your present moment in time, and not in terms of what is potentially natural for a future fully actualized system.

Consequently, the fire systems stress more forceful action, sometimes holding and using forceful breath, muscular contractions, and rigid thoughts about the way things should be done. Conversely, the water schools emphasize letting go, deep mental as well as physical relaxation, softer and continuous breathing without holding the breath, and allowing the Chi of a situation to determine your actions, rather than molding a situation to your will.*

---

*Accordingly, when you view a teacher's instructional demeanor and conversation, you can often determine where his or her bias lies concerning fire and water.

FOCUS ON A SPECIAL TOPIC
The Five Elements:
Reconnecting with Yourself

 Many of the ancient spiritual traditions believe that all manifested sentient and nonliving matter, both on this earth and in the whole universe, is governed and composed of five phases (elements) of energy. The primary energies are in constant flux and each exerts influences on the others. In the Chinese tradition, for example, the five elements are called metal, water, wood, fire, and earth. In the Hindu, yogic, and Buddhist systems they are called space, water, air/wind, fire, and earth. The ancient Western systems deleted one element, leaving four: earth, fire, air, and water.* The ancient traditions held that these five energies, singly or in combination, cause manifestation to occur. When a manifested form loses all cohesion, it reverts back into the unmanifested five energies. The five/four elements were a major component of most ancient meditation and medical systems, especially Taoist-based Chinese medicine and Indian ayurveda. Their goal was to bring the five elements into proper balance for an individual.

What are the relative balances of your own constitution within the five-element theory? The best way to determine it is to seek competent Chinese astrologers, doctors, or meditation adepts who are willing to share their insights with you.

THE FIVE ELEMENTS

Element	Internal organ	Positive emotion	Negative emotion
Metal	Lungs	Happiness/ enthusiasm	Grief/sadness
Water	Kidneys	Vitality	Depression/ fear
Wood	Liver	Compassion/ ability to act	Anger/rage
Fire	Heart	Joy	Anxiety/ overexcitement
Earth	Spleen	Balance/ grounding	Disassociation

*By the Renaissance, the West recognized "ether" or space as a fifth element, or quintessence.

THE WAY OF LIU
Teacher of Two Traditions: Fire and Water Cycles over a Lifetime

Chinese history embraces both the fire and water methods of the Tao. In fact, in both traditions there are the practices of the water and the fire mixing, what is sometimes in Chinese called *kan li lien fa*. The Taoist meditation master Liu Hung Chieh taught me the classical water tradition of Lao Tse.

Before meeting Liu, I practiced many fire methods to great depth. Because it countered the depths of my innate energetic nature I often got hurt physically, emotionally, and psychically; I bulldozed my way through obstacles that could have been bypassed. When I went toward the water technique, obstacles vanished—many of the limitations in my physical and spiritual practices naturally dissolved.

Liu was a conservative Taoist. Though it was difficult, he was a virtual recluse in the middle of Beijing. That was his way. The way he taught me was different, but still within the water tradition. I am very active in the world. So is Liu's only other disciple since China's Communist Revolution in 1949, Bai Hua, who was primarily taught fire practices right from the beginning because Liu could see that Bai Hua's constitution was inclined toward that energy. Liu himself practiced mostly fire methods when younger and the water methods in his later years. This kind of reversal, or rather, completion of an energy cycle, is common as people go through to the opposite from where they started to complete their energetic possibility. If one starts with fire, water completes; if one starts with water, though, it may not be necessary to complete with fire.

The Fire Method Is Based on the Micro/Macrocosmic Orbit of Energy; the Water Method Is Based on Inner and Outer Dissolving

Both the fire and the water methods circulate chi through the same channels, three energy tantiens, meridian lines, points, internal organs, glands, brain centers, blood, and other bodily fluids. Methodologies may differ in their sequences of working the channels, but sooner or later all the channels are more or less accessed.

The biggest difference between the Taoist fire and water approaches is that the fire schools usually base their method from beginning to end on the Great and Small Heavenly Circulation of Energy (also called the Grand/Small Circulation or the Micro/Macrocosmic Orbit of Energy). In fact, there are eleven distinct practices that, combined, compose the Great/Small Circulation.*

The beginning fire practices focus on the Small Circulation and *I* (or *yi*, pronounced "yee" in Chinese) or intention method of visualizing energy as moving from the perineum** up the spine to the top of the head through the governing meridian (which influences all the yang meridians of the body), and returning down the front center line of the body through the nose, heart, navel, and groin back to the perineum through the conception meridian (which influences all the yin meridians of the body). These channels are two of acupuncture's eight extraordinary meridian lines. As the practitioner gets more proficient, the Small Circulation is accomplished by creating, in the lower tantien, tremendous heat and then light, which is circulated through the small orbit. The Great Circulation extends the energy circulation throughout the entire torso, head, arms, and legs.

Intermediate fire practices focus on circulating energy between the inside of the spinal cord and the central channel of energy or between the central channel and the front of the body. The advanced practices concentrate on a number of refinements that ultimately culminate in working purely with the pre-birth central channel. After each of the eleven separate micro/macrocosmic orbits are stabilized, they are

---

*Before I studied in-depth with Liu Hung Chieh, I taught these Heavenly Orbit meditation practices in America and Europe during the 1970s. In the early 1980s I taught them in America, Europe, and China.

**The perineum is the area between the anus and the exterior part of the genitalia.

then used to open up the chi of the body's other energy channels, points, glands, organs, brain centers, blood, and fluids. These in turn are linked back to the Grand Circulation, forging the body into one unbroken, interconnected unit.

The water method in the beginning does not center on the Great/Small Circulation. Instead, it focuses on the downward and outer dissolving process, which allows energy to flow where it previously could not or could do so only weakly. Only after the downward dissolving process is reasonably successful and comfortable to do will the practice of bringing energy up the body be brought into play.* And only after both the downward and upward flows of energy are established separately in the water method of Lao Tse will the Great Circulation process be done as a regular practice, if and when sequentially appropriate. In general, the water method tends to focus more on energy movement within the left, right, and central channels, which are pre-birth patterns that move from deep inside the body outward, rather than the post-birth acupuncture meridian patterns which move from the outside in.** The microcosmic orbit along the governing and conception meridians is popular among traditional Chinese medical practitioners because it follows the acupuncture model so closely.

---

*Ascending energy, which arises from the earth, is responsible for causing phenomena to occur and for transforming (and thereby raising) human beings to a higher energy level than their original genetic capacity would dictate at birth. Descending energy comes down from the cosmos through the human body to the earth. Its purpose is to release all energy the body cannot functionally use. Just as in our body we release unusable toxins downward (for example, feces, urine, sweat, the outbreath), we also release toxic or blocked energy down into the ground. Similarly, the ascending current brings energy up the body in the same way an inbreath goes up our nostrils. If a wire (nerve) is not prepared to take a strong electrical current, some damage can occur—burnout, singeing, shorting out, etc. The downward current clears out the weakness in the wire, creating insulation, to accommodate the ascending current and thus save the nervous system from possible harm.

**By "pre-birth" I am referring to the "channels" or movement of energy that begins in the fertilized egg— a central channel develops, then right and left channels. These stay with us throughout our life cycle. The post-birth acupuncture meridians develop later, during fetal development, and follow an outside-to-inward energy flow.

Intermediate water practice focuses on the inner dissolving technique to clear out all negative or dysfunctional energy in the channels, points, organs, glands, brain centers, blood, and other bodily fluids. Through this process you essentially clear out your first six energy bodies and unify them into a single essence (that is, your being).

When you are fully conscious of your essence and your mind has become still, then the final water method stage of internal alchemy begins. Step by step you transmute your now unified essence to higher and more refined levels of clarity and consciousness until ultimately you merge with the Tao.

The Fire and Water Paths: Feeling, Visualization, and Sound

There are numerous meditation techniques in Taoism. In the water method, the basic processes of inner meditation work are accomplished initially through actual feeling, rather than primarily through visualization work, which is often the way of the fire schools.* All Taoists maintain that you can feel energy just as you can feel concrete objects. The capacity for feeling is intrinsic to life in a heavy gravitational field, such as that of the earth. Taoist tradition holds that discorporeal beings have the ability to see and hear but not feel. Humans, in contrast, live in an extremely condensed energy field and therefore can feel.

The physical body you currently own is the densest of your eight energy bodies (see Chapter 2). Water method Taoists believe that since you exist at this level of density, it is extremely important for you to become comfortable with your body, for your body is all about feeling. The easiest way not to feel things is to disconnect from your body by going strictly into your brain (that is, reside mostly in your seeing-

---

*The word *feeling* here refers to actual physical sensation (as when you touch something) and not emotions or moods.

hearing mind rather than your body) and losing yourself in self-obsessed thoughts.

Water method Taoists believe that after this capacity to feel is established in meditation, you can then move into the techniques that use sound and visualizations. Fire method Taoists work with such techniques right from the start. Taoists in general have extremely refined methods of using mantras and sound frequencies.* They have developed a variety of methods in this area, so that if one of them doesn't work for you, you can achieve the same result using another. You can reach the goal of Taoist water meditation purely through feeling or at later stages through a combination of visualization, sound, and feeling. In the end, after progressive training, what Taoists want is for all the external systems of your body to become completely alive *internally*. By this they mean that you can literally feel everything going on inside yourself, from your liver function to your blood flow to how your emotions, thoughts, and psychic perceptions are affecting the physical tissues of your body in both gross and ever more subtle ways.

---

*A mantra is a specific word or sound that conveys a meaning. By constant repetition with various specific inflections and vibratory distinctions, a mantra has the ability to release a whole series of energies that can manifest on a gross or subtle level. The manifestations can be in the conscious or subconscious mind, in the present or in the future.

The Teacher-Student Relationship in the Fire and Water Approaches

CHAPTER

4

Lao Tse Tao Te Ching, Verses 53 and 81

To know others is intelligence
Knowing yourself is the dawn of genuine wisdom
The mastery of others requires strength
Mastering yourself is true power

The Teacher-Student Relationship in the Fire and Water Approaches

A teacher can hand over to a student only what he or she knows and is able and willing to communicate. There is an old saying in China: "Many who know do not teach. Many who teach do not know. Those who both know and are able to teach are rare indeed." Of the different ways students are taught in Taoism, the most important is by mind-to-mind transmissions.

Mind-to-Mind Transmission

Mind-to-mind transmission is one of the traditional ways that esoteric information has been passed between living persons from generation to generation for thousands of years. In effect, such transmission is a form of telepathy, where one person mentally transmits the totality of a learning experience, including preparation for receiving the learning and integration of the material into the core of the recipient's being, into the receiving individual's very blood and bones, so to speak.*

*_Telepathy_ is the closest English word we have to describe this process, which is not really telepathic in the sense of one person mentally reaching directly into the mind of another to implant, control, or seize thought. It is more on the order of information imbedded in outgoing energy waves that meet and mix with the energy waves of another's mind and somehow effect a transfer of knowledge into the energy field of the other and hence into the mind. The recipient may have to wait for some time to become aware of the teaching, as the transmission behaves like a seed unfolding genetic instruction. The energy generated by the sender is enormous.

Although words and symbolic representations or images can allude to mind/body/spirit knowledge, the words and symbols themselves are rather like the shadow of the thing, rather than the thing itself. With a mind-to-mind transmission, the "whole thing" is directly transmitted to the learner in a holographic form in which the totality of the teacher's knowledge is imparted directly to the student, who must be ready to receive it. Once planted, perhaps to some extent in the student's conscious awareness and, even deeper, in the subconscious mind, the knowledge acts like a time release capsule. As the learner spiritually matures he or she grasps the subtleties of all aspects of what is being learned. The knowledge emerges from the subconscious to full conscious awareness. Mind-to-mind transmission allows the teacher's complete knowledge, realizations, and experience to be transferred to the student without obstruction.

Although the teacher may use highly precise and instructive words, it is the underlying direct and usually silent mind-to-mind transmissions that eventually, if not immediately, allow the student to understand the teachings in their entirety. From this esoteric point of view, teachers cannot teach what they themselves do not truly understand.

Mind-to-mind transmission forms the core of all the traditional teachings about consciousness, not only in Taoism but in all the ancient traditions, including Buddhism, yoga, Sufism, shamanism, and tantra. It is the true message that an authentic guru or yogi gives during satsang/darshan in India, the dharma that a lama or roshi transmits, or, for that matter, how the burning bush spoke to Moses on Mount Sinai. It is for this reason that the words or teachings of a realized adept, or teacher of subtle knowledge, are prized above the mere intellectual scholar who knows the words but lacks the essence that turns dead, dry explanations into living spiritual reality for a living being.

The Teacher-Student Relationship in the Fire Tradition

The Neo-Taoist fire tradition places heavy influence on who is the teacher and who the student, who is the senior student and who the junior. This hierarchy is extremely binding in terms of required responsibilities and obligations between teacher and student or disciple. Much Taoist literature pertaining to immortals, psychic powers, or gods descending to earth to teach spiritual alchemy to ordinary people usually derive from the fire tradition and portray an overt or implied rules-driven relationship between teacher and student.

The fire traditions sometimes did adopt the same position as the water schools of Lao Tse on the student-teacher issue, but more often assumed a point of view similar to other guru-centered mystical traditions and religions. For example, in Indian yogic traditions the guru-disciple relationship is made very clear. Student behavior is highly regulated. You are told in no uncertain terms what to do, how to do it, and how not to do it, and you are chastised overtly and subtly if you do not behave accordingly. To a certain degree, the same is true in Buddhist traditions. With most Buddhist, Sufi, Hindu, and Christian traditions, there is a strong and fixed sense of how a student should relate to the guru, priest, lama, monk, and so on.

FOCUS ON A SPECIAL TOPIC
Recognizing the Problems of Cults
for Both Teachers and Students

At their roots, regardless of philosophical doctrine, all spiritual groups, both East and West, operate somewhere between integrity and manipulation, honesty and sham.

Christianity, currently the world's largest spiritual practice, began as a specific "sect" or "cult" within Judaism two thousand years ago. Although

FOCUS ON A SPECIAL TOPIC
Recognizing the Problems of Cults
for Both Teachers and Students (continued)

Jesus himself was an honest spiritual teacher of integrity, across the centuries other Christian leaders and sects have not always maintained those standards, from the Crusaders who "killed for Christ" to today's charismatic figures who get their followers to commit mass suicide. These conditions hold equally true for meditation and prayer groups, both esoteric and orthodox, whether they believe in God, Christ, Buddha, or the Tao. Fortunately for humanity, spiritual groups lean more toward honesty and integrity as a general rule.

In this book those groups that operate from manipulation, dishonesty, and sham will be called cults, rather than spiritual groups. There will always be a small minority of individuals who become cult leaders to deliberately manipulate and exploit people for their own benefit, just as there will always be the dishonest and corrupt politicians, bureaucrats, and business leaders at every level.

Sincere students and teachers of the Tao who have a strong desire for spiritual clarity need to differentiate between honest spiritual groups with integrity and manipulative cults. For thousands of years Taoists have observed that cults do not spiritually serve either their leaders or followers. Both cult leaders and students can be blithely unaware of the future repercussions of their obvious and hidden motivations and self-delusions.

Many corrupt spiritual leaders, especially those with smaller cults, begin with surface integrity and pure motivations, but over time turn to the dark side for a multitude of reasons. Some never truly learned the genuine inner humility or hard work of being a student. Some became teachers before completing their studies. Now, as their flock's adulation increases, they begin to be influenced by, believe in, and succumb to their students' overt or subtle demands to be manipulated. Sooner or later they run out of genuine teaching material but find they have become attached to and crave the perks of being an adored leader. Rather than humbly admitting that they have no more to teach and saying, "It's time to learn from someone more accomplished," they begin to manipulate their students psychologically in order to maintain their status. Some find that the volume of psychic energy they absorb from their students destabilizes their

FOCUS ON A SPECIAL TOPIC
*Recognizing the Problems of Cults
for Both Teachers and Students (continued)*

inner being, causing them to sink into the deeper and darker sides of their nature faster than they can handle or transmute. Some simply slide down the slippery slopes of self-delusion or choose expediency and the path of least resistance over honesty and integrity.

How do people set themselves up for being exploited by a cult? Students need to ask this question while looking honestly and deeply at their own motivations, in order not to become subject to a cult leader's manipulation. Because the human desire to belong to a group is both powerful and natural, the true motivation of many aspiring spiritual students is to find a social group to belong to, rather than to find a teacher who can genuinely help them to belong to themselves.

Are secular and spiritual goals and needs different? In normal secular society, with its strong social, economic, and political agendas, people often allow external images—physical beauty, clothes, education, way of speaking, class, economic status, and so on—to become powerful motivating forces. For many the primary focus is on style over substance; the cover is more important than the book's contents. Conversely, true students of the Tao should not take any spiritual teacher's externals all that seriously. Rather, a teacher's inner essence, knowledge, and integrity should be the prime concern. A genuine spiritual seeker's focus should be on substance over style.

When students become trapped by externals, the danger exists that they will sooner or later divert their internal efforts away from meditation and into mimicking the teacher's image—possessions, clothes, hairstyle, language, gestures, and so on—becoming "act as if" clones. A good cult leader can manipulate mental or emotional images much more easily than true spiritual substance. If a student's motivations are image oriented, it becomes possible for the cult leader, often using subliminal hypnotic methods, to gradually shift and mold the student's images into extremely convoluted beliefs, which can have dangerous consequences. At the extremes, an image-desiring student is set up to be exploited by unscrupulous gurus or self-deluded crazies.

These cult leaders use and project a multitude of external images to attract different crowds. They are equally likely to wear conventional suits and dresses, embroidered silks, ethnic

FOCUS ON A SPECIAL TOPIC
Recognizing the Problems of Cults
for Both Teachers and Students (continued)

costumes, or robes. They may look, speak, and act like well-groomed salesmen or professors, street hustlers, humble clerics, cryptic kung fu television characters, or Jesus Christ "wannabes" with long hair, beard, and robe, quoting biblical passages most convincingly.

To quote a common saying, misery loves company. The needs of students with psychological weak spots or damaged emotional lives to act out dysfunctionally, be conflicted and indecisive, or have endlessly convoluted relationships with parents and family are often transferred to the teacher and the cult community.

Students should note whether they personally, or the members of the spiritual group or cult they are investigating, allow, encourage, and play these neurotic games. Some individuals misinterpret the idea of a spiritual friend to mean, "Oh boy, now I can mistreat my new spiritual buddies like all my other friends, who mostly tell me to get lost because I act so horribly." This attitude easily opens the door for some enterprising cult leader to brainwash, manipulate, and abuse them in sadly absurd ways. Responsible spiritual teachers will not encourage these mentally unhealthy relationship games and will maintain distance from those that do, as these spiritually corrosive games breed neurosis and easily escalate into the danger zone.

Good teachers encourage relaxed relationships and cooperation between spiritually inclined individuals, not conflict. Students of the Tao endeavor to treat spiritual friends well, with respect, and with honest, open agendas. Taoists consider these hallmarks of spiritually productive teacher-student relationships. Taoists believe it is good not to confuse human relationships predicated upon compassion, balance, and integrity with those based on the need to defend self-aggrandizing ego tendencies and hidden agendas about power and control that imprison the spirit. Chains, whether made of steel or gold, still bind.

The Teacher-Student Relationship in the Water Tradition

The Taoists of the water tradition believe that if individuals have genuinely decided to develop their essence, then they are automatically pointed in the direction to reach that end. There is no need to continuously remotivate them.

The water tradition of China embraces the marvelous idea that all are friends in the Tao, and that natural respect comes from deep inside the mind and heart. The outer show of it is not such a big deal; consequently, demonstrations of respect follow normal lines rather than formal bows, hand positions, or kowtows. The water tradition is neither rigid nor formal.

In those instances where their students fail to grant them respect, water tradition teachers are likely to just shrug their shoulders and gently avoid engaging with the student concerning serious subjects. Their attitude is that such disrespect is not much different from the behavior of a child who doesn't know any better. The teacher will wait until the student matures and comes to realize that, contrary to the old saying "familiarity breeds contempt," water method Taoists believe that familiarity and informality breed respect.

Historically, Taoist teachers deliberately discourage more often than entice prospective students. Once a water tradition teacher detects genuine resolve in a student, though, the feeling is that, no matter how many zigzags it takes, the student will ultimately reach the Tao. It may take a day, a week, a year, a million years, but that student is eventually going to get there. The road the student is on *is* the Tao, which is changeless and beyond influence. At the end of the day, you will be with friends practicing the Tao together. Knowing that this bond of respect for the Tao exists in both student and teacher, Taoist masters of the water method tend to treat their students as friends rather than as underlings, even though at this point in time the masters are more developed spiritually. They want their students to decide for themselves how to live, what to learn, how much to practice, and so forth. They want to create fully independent spiritual beings.

THE WAY OF LIU
The Decision to Teach

      My teacher Liu Hung Chieh was a water-
method person. The water method is all I practice now. Having been immersed in the fire
method for many years, and in youth having
practiced both the Zen tradition in America
and Japan and the tantric and kundalini tradi-
tions in India, I went on to learn the Taoist fire tradition in
Taiwan and Hong Kong, where it is difficult to find the water
tradition. When I reached a point where the fire tradition no
longer satisfied me, the water tradition found me. I was not
particularly looking for the water tradition—it found me.
There was no intent on my part.

During my seven years in Taiwan and Hong Kong, I did
much of the fire method's introductory energy channel work
and a great deal of sexual meditation work. I was fortunate
to be trained as a fully empowered Taoist priest (taoshr)
during those years. I learned arts such as exorcism, sending
people off when they die, empowerment, and charging
spaces (such as temples or practice spaces). This was my
preparation for studying in Beijing with my main teacher,
Liu Hung Chieh, from whom I learned the real water tradition in depth.

I was extremely fortunate to study with Liu. Frankly
speaking, this did not come about through any good efforts
of my own, but rather because Liu had had a dream about a
foreigner coming to him right before I arrived. I became one
of only two students (and the only Westerner) that he taught
comprehensively after the Communists rose to power in
1949.

Almost a year before Liu died, he began to encourage me
to teach Taoism and Taoist meditation when I returned to the
West. At first I felt uncomfortable with that prospect, feeling
that I did not know enough to do so, or even if I did, I didn't
feel the time was right yet. During the last year that he was
alive, 1986, Liu said, "If you are willing to teach, do it; if not,
don't bother." It has only been since 1992 that I started
publicly teaching the Taoist water method meditation techniques I learned from Liu.

In the water tradition, if you are able to study with one of the elderly masters (the literal translation of the name Lao Tse is "old one"), consider yourself lucky, for you are with someone who has pretty much mastered what is inside of him or her. Be quiet and respectful. Listen, learn, and practice. Grace and respect will allow your spiritual flowering to proceed at the smoothest and most rapid pace. In this manner the younger Taoists in the water tradition place great emphasis, not on the superior master/inferior disciple construct, but on the inner connection between master and disciple. That is the nature of love.

How a Student Should Relate to a Teacher/Adept in Taoism

Sometimes, students of spirituality have image and attitude problems regarding their teachers, holding expectations impossible for the teacher to fulfill. Such students often overtly or subtly demand that their teacher should look and act like an idealized image of what a "spiritual master" should be or the role model of what they, the students, wish to buy. What is really important, however, is the teacher's practical knowledge of meditative techniques and the workings of Consciousness, and the teacher's ability to impart that knowledge.

Teachers with integrity seek students uninterested in projecting godhead on them. They tend to work with individuals serious about concentrating on their internal activity, about balancing their bodies, opening their energy channels, making their emotions clear and nonreactive, and stilling their hearts and minds. Genuinely competent teachers may not be "politically correct." They will, though, say what they mean and do what they say. Good teachers are looking for good students, as much as if not more than the other way around.

The perspective of teachers in Taoism is that of someone who will lend you spiritual power and wisdom, but who will demand that you keep your power and increase it in your own way and own time. Taoism focuses on the individual, not the group. The goal of Taoist teachers is to help students eventually become their spiritual equals. To this end, they recognize that both the teacher and the student must exercise patience, balance, and forbearance, so that student and teacher do not make spiritual fools of

THE WAY OF LIU
A Teacher-Student Relationship

     In the unbalanced exuberance of youth, I told Liu I wanted "to be just like him." He stared at me silently for a long time, then looked me right in the eye and began to laugh. When he finished, he said, "Really? It would be useful and valuable for you to wish to develop your consciousness, but do you really want to lose the enjoyment of fine food, beautiful women, seeing the world, only to live alone meditating all day? Would you really like to have lived under Communism for over thirty years and have experienced the sadness of the Cultural Revolution?" He then told me, "I am me and you are you. There is no need for you to give up your internal freedom to be like me, or me to give up my internal freedom to make you feel better. Let us focus on your work at hand—making your consciousness free. Emulate my consciousness, not my personality. You have the right to your own unique expression; you need not be an imitation of mine. In this way, both our freedoms will not be trapped by mutual admiration and control. My job as a spiritual teacher is to help you find your spiritual heart, power, and clarity, not to control you with mine. I am unwilling to allow myself to be controlled by your need to worship a god so you can dodge the effort of working on yourself."

I voiced the ancient words that sprang to my mind: "If you do not wish to be someone's slave, do not become a master." Liu agreed. He said, "Masters do not act the true way of their integrity because they are afraid they will produce an image that the slaves will revolt against, thereby stripping them of their privileges. Likewise, slaves do not take responsibility for their being, because they just obey and give all responsibility and the hard, difficult choices of life, which demand growing into maturity, over to their masters."

themselves but eventually, in collaboration, can help balance all under the Tao.

Dangers Inherent in All Manipulative Cults

In stark contrast to the traditionally honored position of a teacher and student in water method Taoism is the spiritually contorted situation of a manipulating cult leader and his or her followers. Taoism discovered thousands of years ago (and has reaffirmed to the present) that the teacher's wisdom should be used to "give back" students' innate power to themselves so they can become spiritually clear. The teacher only sparingly, if at all, uses power to control the neurotic, immoral, or unconscious impulses of students, and then usually only out of genuine compassion to stop them metaphorically from falling off a dangerous cliff they do not know is there. Most of the time the teacher will not interfere. A good teacher knows it is better for students to get singed by danger and learn their lesson, rather than be unnecessarily rescued from a minor burn only to be left still unaware, so they can be spiritually burned alive in a really dangerous situation, when the teacher is not there to help them. The object of the true Taoist teacher is like the parents of a bird: to get the newborns out of the nest, flying on their own as soon as possible.

The agenda of cult leaders is different. They want their followers to become totally dependent on them, to believe that without the teacher's "something," the student will never make it on his or her own. In other words, cult leaders want to addict disciples to the leader's presence, words, appearance, community, and psychic energy. Bai Hua, Liu's other student and my teacher for many years, once likened this situation to the relationship of a totally unempowered baby who sees the solution to everything in life in the sweet milk of its mother's breast. On this basis, it is impossible for the student to become spiritually mature and independent.

Cult leaders want this dependence. They want control over your power either to enhance ego, worldly pleasures, money, and secular power, or to feed their unbalanced inner compulsions. Taoism has watched cults come and go for millennia. It is clear that the cult mentality can pervert the natural wisdom and relationship of trust between a teacher and student. Genuine students should look within to be certain that they are not seeking to be controlled by a teacher in order to satisfy some inner need. Genuine teachers also should not be drawn into the psychological problems of students out of a natural desire to help. Both teachers and students should be aware of the issue of transference. Many cults are only too happy to take "lost souls" and recondition or exploit them, psychologically and financially. In doing so, cult leaders often use tools such as playing upon emotions or guilt, convincing students to turn over assets, promising great "secret powers," encouraging spiritual and secular greed, and requiring arcane rules of behavior and ritualistic action. There should be no demand—from anyone—that students be clones of their teachers.

How a Genuine Spiritual Teacher Helps an Aspiring Student

There are genuine rewards for working with an honest, skilled, and compassionate spiritual guide. There are also potential pitfalls to finding and working with any teacher. As mentioned, teachers come in good, incompetent, wise, self-deluded, honest, and unethical sizes.

When you enter into a spiritual journey, you frequently have no idea where you are and what is happening. You may feel lost in a vast expanse, without landmarks or map. Disoriented, you lose track of where you have been and are insecure about how to proceed. Genuine spiritual teachers can help you get your bearings. They have already been there, know the territory, and have successfully crossed it. They see the whole view, while you may only see disconnected fragments.

The valuable, reliable, and experienced wisdom such teachers can offer may or may not be obvious to you. They can, however, help you to (a) learn when to have confidence in your intuitions; (b) recognize when psychological problems are getting in the way; and (c) avoid or mitigate self-delusion and other mental traps (or at least not make them worse than they need to be). Authentic teachers of spirituality will not abuse your trust.

The Importance of Respect and Integrity in the Teacher-Student Relationship

Taoists value human feeling, respect, and integrity. If the bonds of mutual human affection are absent, the teacher-student relationship can easily become unbalanced. Both parties may then be tempted to use the relationship for their own profit or private agenda and may no longer wish to put energy into the work. In the natural course of human interactions, misunderstandings and grievances invariably pop up. During trying times, forgiveness and forbearance are essential for continuing productive interactions between people of good faith. However, it is the student who must want to stay with the teacher. A genuinely nonattached Taoist teacher will leave a door open to students but will not play games to get them back. If the bond of human affection gets deeply frayed, though, either party may not go the extra mile to work things out.

Respect, especially for the Tao itself, is in many ways even more important for the Taoist teacher than is human affection. If students do not respect a teacher's accomplishment and/or sincerity in teaching meditation, they should not spend time with that teacher. Legitimate teachers who do not respect their students' integrity will not spend effort on them. What is being imparted transcends the self-interest of both the teacher and the student. Such work requires honesty and respect for it to bear fruit.

Teachers will sometimes push students extremely hard. Sometimes, out of frustration, students then behave disrespectfully toward the teacher. The student should make

FOCUS ON PRACTICE
Taoist Internal Breathing, Lesson 6

- We are now going, in stages, to continue the awareness of breath down to just below the navel.
- Begin with 2 breaths. With each, on the inhale, continue the awareness of your breath from your nose through the center of your body down to the bottom of your chest. Without breaking your conscious awareness of your breath, on the exhale follow your breath back up your chest, to your throat, and through and out your nose. Keep trying until you can do this without a break in your awareness.
- Next, with continuous awareness and body feeling, follow the inhaled breath from your nose to your throat through the center of your body to the bottom of your chest, down to the middle of your stomach, and on the exhale, back up to your chest, throat, and out your nose.
- Inhale downward through your nose, throat, and chest, ending at your navel. Retrace the same path on the exhale. Practice 2 breaths, rest, and continue over and over again until you can do so with a relaxed body and mind in a comfortable way with continuous awareness.
- Continue your inhalation (from nose to navel), breathing downward to the middle of your belly, about half the distance between your navel and pubic hair. The Chinese call this location the lower tantien. Practice until you can breath down to the lower tantien with uninterrupted concentration, feeling, and awareness in a continuous, comfortable, and relaxed fashion both mentally and physically for 2 complete breaths.
- Expand to 3 breaths, then 4, then to 1 complete set of 10 breaths.
- Increase to 2 sets of 10, then 3, then 4, then 5 complete sets of 10 breaths.
- This exercise will significantly increase both your ability to feel the inside of your body and the strength of your conscious awareness.

every effort not to do so. Disrespect can cut off the wellspring a teacher requires to do the work properly. For students to express what their innermost needs are is fine; disrespectful behavior displayed in words, deeds, or attitudes is not. Taoist teachers often do not demand strong external shows of respect, such as bowing, genuflection, specific titles, or formal behaviors. However, both in human demeanor and heartfelt sincerity, without the respect of the student, the teacher cannot fully open up.

As the student perseveres and demonstrates appreciation for the Tao and for meditation, the teacher will watch closely to see if integrity is evidenced. If it is, and the teacher finds nothing personally offensive about the student, their relationship might progress from being polite strangers to being spiritual friends.

Not All Meditation Experiences Mean That Something Is Afoot

About 95 percent of the internal experiences that spiritual practice generates are no more than the natural releasing and cleansing of the "stuff" inside the human psyche. No more than 5 percent of those internal experiences have significant implications for the practitioner.

A good teacher can see what is going right and what is going wrong for you, or can show you how to move and progress in a direction you would not have thought of by yourself. The teacher can guide you through dangerous reefs and help you to understand the context of your meditative experiences.

Besides helping their students to avoid traps, maximize practice time, and make use of spontaneously arising positive opportunities, teachers also keep a watchful eye out for those in their tutelage who may fall victim to spiritual drift or lethargy. When you as a student sink into states such as these, a teacher is invaluable for setting you straight so you don't waste time in a quagmire. Real teachers want to empower you to recognize the difference between your true inner voice and any self-deluding internal garbage, including mental drift, meaning a state of confused ambiguity.

Correcting Bad Spiritual Habits and Instilling Good Ones

Many students who accumulate partial spiritual awareness and power become arrogant with a false sense of superiority, display contempt for "lesser beings" (including their teachers and fellow students), lose a sense of compassion, and end up as self-aggrandizing monsters. A teacher is then obliged to encourage such a student to confront this behavior. Some wild beast egos are best tamed with a gentle hand, and some respond best to forceful attention. A good teacher needs to be compassionate and balanced enough to respond flexibly to the changing modes of students during the meditative journey.

Even more important, a competent teacher expends effort to instill good spiritual habits and values in students, always encouraging them to cultivate balance, compassion, generosity, wisdom, and empathy, and to have the strength to do what must be done and the strength to leave alone that which needs to be left alone. Humans, including teachers, are not perfect. Taoists believe that it is from the fertile soil of respect, generosity, and wisdom that the Tao can naturally grow. The Taoist perspective for thousands of years has been that if an accomplished spiritual teacher is willing and able to apply the Golden Rule to students, the students are the recipients of rare good fortune.

Taoist Meditation:
An Overview

CHAPTER
5

Lao Tse Tao Te Ching, Verse 15

*Can you find the patience to wait
Until your dust settles
And the water becomes clear?*

Taoist Meditation: An Overview

When you start to learn Taoist meditation, your first six bodies (physical, chi, emotional, mental, psychic, and causal) are in confusion, like dust in a glass of swirling water. Both your personal consciousness and Universal Consciousness itself are hidden by the stirred mud of confused Chi. The murkiness is often thick enough to cause a loss of your inner stability and sense of cohesion. You do not have sufficient internal focus present to support a strong self-image or to clear away all the supercharged emotional and traumatic ghosts from your personal past. Yet such clearing is a prerequisite for being aware of your own consciousness, let alone Universal Consciousness.

A journey of a thousand miles begins with a single step. Each step thereafter should be taken only when the preceding one has been completed, or you will likely trip, possibly hurting yourself. So it is with Taoist meditation. First of all, the preparatory physical and chi practices clear, balance, and energize your distorted first six bodies.

Preparatory (Beginning) Practices

The aim of the beginning practices is to develop an awareness of subtle energy in your body and to maintain that awareness. The benefits of the beginning practices include improved health, vitality, calmness, and the awareness necessary for the middle practices.

Diagram B

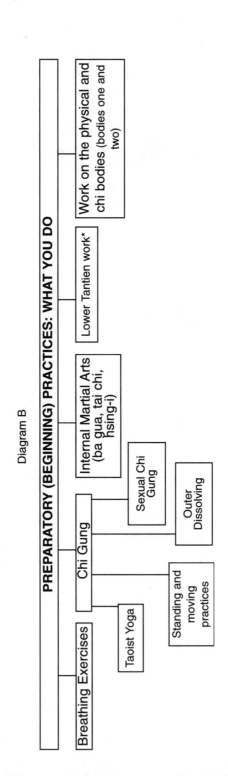

PREPARATORY (BEGINNING) PRACTICES: WHAT YOU DO

- Breathing Exercises
  - Taoist Yoga
- Chi Gung
  - Standing and moving practices
  - Sexual Chi Gung
  - Outer Dissolving
- Internal Martial Arts (ba gua, tai chi, hsing-i)
- Lower Tantien work*
- Work on the physical and chi bodies (bodies one and two)

*There are three main tantiens (pronounced "dandiens"), or energy centers, in the human body. These are the places where chi collects and governs a person's energetic anatomy. The lower tantien, located just below the navel in the center of the body, is the energetic center primarily responsible for the health of the human body and the only center where all the energies that affect the physical body interact. The middle tantien has two locations: at the solar plexus and at the center of the chest near the heart (we will refer to this latter location as the middle tantien throughout the book). The first governs the functions of the middle internal organs; the second governs relationships with sentient beings. The upper tantien, located in the brain, controls human perceptual mechanisms and psychic functions.

THE WAY OF LIU
Liu Explains the Process of Meditation

In his beginning teachings, Liu Hung Chieh explained the meditation process to me this way: He took a glass of clear water and said that this water is like a human being's original nature (individual essence) before confusion separated it from both itself and the Tao. This clear water is also what we all are going to evolve to and return to sooner or later. He then mixed some reddish dirt into the glass and stirred it. This dirt, he said, is like all the energies (karma)* that surround and are attached to you, confuse and disconnect you from your essence, and keep you from experiencing yourself as your essence. We confuse the red dust with our intrinsic Consciousness and falsely experience the dust as being the core of our being. This red dust of physical body, chi, emotions, conscious thoughts, psychic perceptions, and causal awareness weakens, obscures, and unbalances our lives.

Liu set the glass of swirling water down and we watched the dust move. The settling of the dust, he said, represents the beginning process of Taoist meditation, where the meditator dissolves blockages in his or her physical body, chi, and emotions. Just when the dust began to settle almost completely to the bottom of the glass, and the water was almost clear, Liu stirred it up again. Meditating, he said, is just like this. Often, just when you feel clear, more in your unexplored depths is strongly released, the same way the dust exploded up from the bottom of the glass. He said to expect and embrace this frustrating situation, which is part of human nature. Liu said everyone wants quick success. Yet it is only the road of patience and diligence that can ultimately leave a human being deeply satisfied. In meditation, that which does not allow the water to taste absolutely sweet is the dust-filled content of your energies and mind.

We watched many stirrings and settlings together. Finally, Liu allowed the dust to rest at the bottom of the glass. The water was now pristine and clear. Liu explained that this

---

*Karma is the Buddhist and Hindu religious concept that asserts that all the memories, impressions, attachments, aversions, and tendencies of your current and past lives are imbedded in your soul. These powerful influences naturally activate when certain circumstances in your life occur, greatly affecting you.

THE WAY OF LIU
Liu Explains the Process of Meditation (continued)

distinct separation of the dust and the water signifies the dawning stage of emptiness and emotional maturity. When, through meditation, you reach this point in your awareness, you become able to realize the emptiness that was symbolized by the water. Liu said that, at this juncture, the meditator has to practice for a while to stabilize this level of mind, which can recognize emptiness, always a most difficult feat. If the glass is not kept still through meditation, the water can again become muddy. Consequently, he said, it is mandatory to practice regularly in order to prevent the dust from swirling once more, confusing everything.

Liu then said that I had to decide what my motivation for meditating was all about, in order to determine if it was even useful to move on to discussing the next stage, internal alchemy. I asked him what he meant. He explained that the emotional maturity practice is sufficient for gaining success in the martial and healing arts, as well as achieving reasonably balanced emotions and peace of mind. However, a meditator who has succeeded in merely separating the dust and the water has insufficient skills to complete his or her spiritual evolution and to fully become one with the Tao. Using Buddhist concepts, Liu said there was still all the past karma to be reckoned with, that which the individual had accumulated before being born. The red dust collected at the bottom of the glass now has to be dissolved.

Liu described this dissolving as the beginning of internal alchemy, the concluding stage of Tao practices. Here, Liu maintained, the dust has to be dissolved and transmuted many times so that after a while it distracts you less and less from your individual essence. After alchemical work, all the dust will be gone and only the water will remain. At this point the meditator can clearly identify both dust and water for what they are and were. When you have reached this stage, Liu said, you can begin the first day of true meditation—the previous work essentially having been only introductory practices concerned with distortions of reality. From here on, you have to keep meditating or new dust from events that occur in the world can again come into your "glass," your conscious awareness. Now the dissolving process begins again, this time dissolving and refining the emptiness that is the water itself, until the water is

THE WAY OF LIU

Liu Explains the Process of Meditation (continued)

transmuted into the stuff of the Tao itself. This follows the classic Taoist formula (as shown in Chapter 2) of:

jing (physical body) transforms to
Chi (energy), which transforms to
shen (spirit), which transforms to
wu (emptiness; Consciousness; the clear water with
dust on the bottom), which transforms to
the Tao or the Way (only water).

Our conversation on this subject occurred in 1981. Liu proclaimed that I had reached the decision point: it was time to decide whether or not to make a commitment to the difficult task of taking on spiritual evolution. He repeated that this was going to be harder than learning the martial and healing arts combined and emphasized that it had to be my own decision. Unlike other traditions, Taoists do not feel it is right to influence or interfere with an individual's complete freedom of choice in such an ultimately important matter. Liu reminded me that I could consider this decision at some other time in the future, if in the depth of my heart I felt that it might not be the right time to decide now. There was no rush. I replied that discovering the Tao was more important to me than the martial arts or healing arts, both of which I deeply loved. Thus I began to study Taoist meditation and later internal alchemy with Liu until he died on December 1, 1986. True to Liu's word, the work was the most formidable, yet the most fulfilling, that I had ever encountered in my life. Since then, my personal work with internal alchemy has been ongoing.

FOCUS ON PRACTICE
Taoist Internal Breathing, Lesson 7

You should now be able to maintain a line of awareness from your nose through the center of your body to your lower tantien. From here on, do your best to completely relax your chest and not use any strength in your chest or puff it out when you breathe.

- Let the feeling of the center line inside your body (where your central channel is located), from the middle of your throat to lower tantien, expand forward and backward until you can feel the whole inside of your belly, micro-inch by micro-inch. Now think of your belly as a cylinder and use your breath to expand it equally in all directions from its center line—forward, backward, and equidistant out to the sides.
- In the beginning, focus on the easiest movement, which is that of the lower belly. When this is comfortable, turn your attention to add the more difficult movement of the middle belly. Finally, concentrate on and add the most difficult part of the body to gain control of—the solar plexus and diaphragm.
- Now as you follow the awareness of your breath from your nose to tantien,
    1. On your inbreath, feel your belly expanding from your center line *forward* to the skin on the front of your body. On the outbreath, return your belly to its original position.
    2. Now on the inbreath, expand the inside of your body *backward* from your center line to your spine. On the exhale, relax your body to its original position.
    3. On the inhale, from the center line of the body expand *backward* and *forward* at the same time, both toward the skin on the front of your belly and your spine. On the exhale, return to your original position.
- The simultaneous backward and forward motion is what you want to achieve. Begin with 2 breaths and rest. After your awareness

FOCUS ON PRACTICE
Taoist Internal Breathing, Lesson 7 (continued)

is continuous, both in and out and to front and back, increase 1 breath at a time with completely relaxed continuity, to 10 and then 15 and then 20 breaths.
- If you lose awareness or space out, start over from the beginning. Day by day you will find the strength of your awareness increasing.

Initially, these preparatory practices are focused on developing your energy channels to have the strength and stability to deal with releasing your repressed emotions with a minimum of shocks or aftershocks. Doing these practices, you prepare for and begin to experience the emotional distortions hidden within yourself. In the course of ordinary life, these emotionally repressed time bombs often erupt at crisis points, such as death, divorce, disease, mid-life crisis, or financial disaster. The preparatory chi practices slow down the emotional swirling of the dust, gradually building internal stability, perception, and calmness until you clearly recognize and accept your difficulties and dysfunction (that is, the dust) for what they are, without self-delusion or denial.

Next, you begin the second stage of meditation practice, the road to maturity and stillness, by learning how to quiet the dissolving dust, clearing out and neutralizing your highly charged positive and negative attachments, past traumas, and internal demons, all of which diminish you and rob you of Chi. After dissolving the distortions and neutralizing them over a considerable period of time, you begin to get flashes of Consciousness (that is, the water) itself, glimpses still mostly clouded with the distortions of your physical, chi, emotional, mental, psychic, and causal bodies.

When your most horrific inner demons have been tamed and you have accomplished emotional and mental well-being and have progressed toward emotionally maturity, it is time to decide if you actually want to take on the task of recognizing Consciousness itself. The water and dust have ceased swirling violently, and the dust particles are now moving in some kind of suspension that allows an inkling that there may indeed be water in the glass. The question then arises: Do I want to discover what this water is? Or was I only interested in a little meditative experience to reduce my stress and get physically and emotionally healthier?

You now have two choices. If your primary goal was to procure physical and emotional health and restore the fractured parts of your identity, then stay with this goal without thinking you need to go any further. Just continue on with the earlier practices of your choice to keep the dust from swirling again. If, however, you want to discover the nature of your spiritual center and Consciousness, then the dissolving process must grow and intensify. Meditation becomes less casual and more serious.

Now you apply the dissolving process to deeper levels until you work at clearing out all your bodies from the physical to the psychic. You then begin to perceive, and for the first time obtain, the capacity to work with and clear out your causal body. As you dissolve and release the glitches in the sixth body, you become empowered to eventually receive the grace that allows you to recognize Consciousness itself. You now begin to experience Consciousness more and more as you progressively become comfortable entering into and stabilizing all the various states of emptiness.

The water of Consciousness is now in slow suspension. Sometimes you can glimpse it between the suspended particles. Through continual dissolving, you may get "peak experiences" or tremendous insights. Your inner voice will be getting clearer all the time, although the danger still exists of confusing it with the voices of your neuroses. Gradually, the previously swirling water dramatically slows. Inner stillness is growing strongly within you.

Then, one day, through deliberate effort, grace, or serendipity, your mind slows and your spirit becomes extremely stable. The dust drops to the bottom of the glass; the swirling motion has stopped. From then on you experience the water—Consciousness itself—as being completely independent of your personality. Your mind becomes still and the goals of the Taoist maturity practices are accomplished. You arrive at the Great Stillness.

You are now—and with practice will continue to be—aware of how living Consciousness activates and defines you, bringing whatever you are engaged in to full life. You also become clear when and how Consciousness is alive within you. You now see and understand the differences between Consciousness, the "water," and your internal conditionings and tendencies, the "red dust." Before this realization, you may have had visions, hopes, or insubstantial intellectual ideas and beliefs about Consciousness, but you were incapable of separating the water and the dust. Now you can.

The spiritual problem of the human ego's incessant need to feel good or always be right has been solved. Like the sun in the sky, you, being fully aware of your individual essence, do not have a need to feel good, only to be. From the point of view of the water school of Taoism, genuine spiritual work (that is, becoming one with the Tao) now begins. For without knowing deeply and personally what Consciousness is, you cannot get beyond beliefs and fear.

You now are like a newborn spiritual infant, newly aware, with the opportunity to grow into a spiritual adult. You can now begin the work of transforming the dust particles at the bottom of the glass into Consciousness through the practice of internal alchemy.* You must always bear in mind, though, that life circumstances can set the dust swirling again if you do not maintain your dissolving practices. You have to keep at it.

---

*Internal alchemy practices are described in volume 2 of this Water Method of Taoist Meditation series, *The Great Stillness.*

FOCUS ON PRACTICE
Taoist Internal Breathing, Lesson 8

The focus is now on breathing beneath the lower ribs.

- On the inhale, physically move and expand the insides of your belly toward the front and sides. Feel the breath move beneath the lower ribs to stimulate your liver on the right side and your spleen on the left.
- On the exhale let your belly return to its original relaxed position.
- Gradually build your breath up with continuous awareness from 2 to 20 breaths.
- Initially put your hands on your sides to physically test if your sides are moving, until without physical touch your awareness alone can tell if your sides are moving or not.

The Standing Mode of Taoist Practice

The Taoist meditation practices taught in both volumes of this book may be done in any of five modes: standing, moving, sitting, lying down, or during sexual activity. The Taoist water tradition, as described in Chapter 3, generally recommends a progression that begins with the standing practices and gradually progresses to moving, then sitting, and then lying down practices. Sexual meditation methods may be practiced as an adjunct to any of the other types, with different sexual methods used at different stages. The present volume deals exclusively with the first two modes, standing and moving; the more advanced practices are discussed in the second volume.

Each practice serves as a firm foundation for the one following, and each must be mastered in turn for its full potential to be actualized. Each practice requires more subtlety, clarity of mind, strength, and stability of awareness than the one before it. Each one requires the mindstream (described later in this chapter) to rely on itself, without any support, while staying focused, aware, and engaged (as opposed to becoming dull or sleepy or numb). Consequently, each successive practice is more powerful than the one preceding it. Remember that this book is designed to be a primer for beginners. As such, it would be inappropriate to include any instructions for the more advanced practices in any mode.

Of the five modes, standing practice is the easiest. Its primary aim is to make the energy of the body healthy, strong, open, and clear, to open energy channels, and to calm the agitation that a tense body and central nervous system produces. As the body stands motionless, every physical imbalance and weakness will reveal itself as the seconds tick by and gravity weighs heavier and heavier. Discomfort, gravity, and the naturally activated automatic reflexes creating the desire not to fall down will sharpen your awareness.

Standing Meditation Exercise

1.   Stand still.
      Your feet should be parallel, about shoulder width apart, arms dangling at your sides, palms facing backward. Relax your breath. Concentrate on your breath and feel its changing qualities. Is your mind calm, still, and comfortable, or is it uneasy and agitated? The whole time you stand, continue to be aware of your breath and feel how your body is changing. Note carefully how your breath goes in and out your nose. Let your breathing deepen, until it becomes slow, steady, and from the belly (see p. 108). Keep the tip of your tongue on the roof of your mouth. Relax any tension in your jaw until it relaxes and drops down, without your mouth opening.

2.   Mentally feel your body from head to toe.

Once your breath becomes stable and you feel yourself consciously aware of your body, go inside with your mind and let your awareness begin to flow from the top of your head downward, equally on the front, back, and sides of your body. First scan along the surface of your skin, then deep into your muscles, and eventually down through your bones. Let your awareness go slowly down your body, spending some time on each area before proceeding to the next blocked point below.

By internally scanning for and actually feeling the sensations in your body, you will gradually become aware of those places where you have tension, blocked strength, contractions, pain, anxiety, or other things that don't feel quite right, especially if you don't know what they are. Continue scanning downward until you reach the bottom of your feet and have relaxed your body sufficiently so you really feel your feet on the ground.

3.   Institute chi-cultivating body alignments.*

Separate your thighs so your perineum feels open and unconstricted. Now bend your knees a couple of inches, making sure they do not extend beyond your toes. Relax the muscles of your lower back and hips, then tuck your pelvis slightly forward while relaxing it toward the ground, without letting your knees bend any farther. Keep your head slightly lifted. Make certain your head does not bend or tilt forward, backward, to the left, or to the right. These alignments will help your body avoid needlessly blocking or dissipating your chi. As you institute these internal body alignments become aware of how, when you gently relax into

---

*For a more complete description of the standing meditation practice outlined here, including full details and illustrations of the correct body alignments, see B. K. Frantzis, *Opening the Energy Gates of Your Body* (Berkeley, Calif.: North Atlantic Books, 1993), Chapters 3 and 4.

a body alignment, the quality of your attention changes. Are your body alignments enhancing or distorting your ability to have a calm, clear mind?

4.   Release all your tension and strength to the ground.

With your full intention, slow your mind down and allow it to observe both itself and your body simultaneously. Then, beginning from the top of your head, let all of your tension and strength internally release and fall downward—toward the ground, and eventually through your body and into the ground—all the while keeping your head properly aligned at the same level.

Notice how releasing tension from your body can also release tension from your thoughts. Often, when our central nervous system is overloaded and we feel stressed out, the place where the stress is lodged in our bodies feels strong. In reality, the feeling of strength and blocked energy are very similar. Release all your strength and tension down to the ground bit by bit. All the while keep your spine straight, head upright, and pelvis tucked under so your tailbone points to the floor. The goal here is eventually to feel the sensation of having energy falling through your legs right into your feet and then into the ground. Again, your knees should not move forward in space past your toes. Your energy should fall *through* the knees, but your knees should not physically fall forward. Your weight should be felt in your calves and feet, not in your knees. The weight passes through the knees to the feet.

When releasing only a part of the body, lightly release all your energy to the ground at the end of the practice session. Spend a week releasing only as far down as your neck. Then spend another week releasing only your head and chest. The next week add the belly. The next week, the head, chest, belly, and pelvic area. The next week, all those plus the legs, all the way down to your feet. And after that, release all your tension and strength, all the way from the head to the feet and into the ground itself. The more you practice, the more your body and mind will relax and be at ease.

5.   Have reasonable expectations.

As you stand, you will slowly begin to feel in fine detail where and how your body is out of balance. By releasing your tension, you will feel much better. The deadened, hard, tense, and uncomfortable spots of your body will become soft, comfortable, and fully alive again. Your blood circulation will improve. The more you practice, the more any neck, shoulder, and back discomfort will disappear. You should feel more open in every joint of your body and taller as your body opens from the inside. To the extent you feel your body dropping and relaxing, you proportionately feel and make your spine rise. As above, so below. The more you fall, the more you rise, and the more you rise, the more you fall.

Standing gives you a reliable way to release the tension accumulated during the day from your body, enabling you to enjoy what's left of your day. For example, you will become aware of where and how you carry tension in your neck, shoulders, back, or any other body part. You will directly experience how deep exhaustion from stress has permeated your body. You may even recognize how your back or hips are going out of alignment, days or weeks before you need to visit a chiropractor, so you can take remedial action before a small problem becomes a big one.

Gradually, the standing practice will demonstrate to you what your natural tension limits are. Usually, most of us are quite unaware of how deeply stress has penetrated our bodies, until extreme pain sets in. Many who practice standing meditation regularly learn what it means to be fully relaxed, for every bit of tension to leave the muscles. By releasing the tensions of the body and mind, you get stronger and are better able to fight off disease.

What Is the Mindstream?

In learning Taoist internal breathing, you have begun to use proprioception (feeling what's happening inside your body) to sharpen your conscious awareness, as a preparation for meditation. The next stage, the standing meditation exercise just described, requires that you become aware of that very awareness. In many meditation traditions, this process is called "the witnessing mind." The witnessing mind just observes what is naturally arising without judgment. It lets the content of events come and go without your influencing them or being influenced by them. Meditators must reach this state of mind, engage with it, and stabilize in it for some period of time. To achieve this ability is an accomplishment in itself. However, it is only the beginning of the meditative process.

As you become more familiar with the process of being aware of awareness itself, you may also begin to sense a subtle stream that pervades your awareness. This is the *mindstream*, the contact point that will eventually lead you to Universal Consciousness itself, which is much greater than mere ordinary awareness. Following and working with the mindstream will eventually take you from the "witnessing mind" to an unbroken sensitivity, to the content attached to your Consciousness, to an awareness of Consciousness itself. According to most if not all of the world's mystic traditions, the mindstream is naturally present in all living creatures, rather than something that needs to be created or embellished.

This mindstream, which is quite distinct from the motion of the mind (going from one conscious thought to the next) is hidden to most of us only because it has never been explicitly sought or given full attention. We normally are so occupied with keeping our attention on the external events of life that we do not even consider the value of this most subtle internal "water" of life. As you emerge more deeply into the mindstream, things that were heretofore incredibly subtle and barely discernible become obvious. This process, in turn, opens up your ability to become aware of the next level of subtlety, previously hidden. Within the mindstream is included, in ever more subtle shades, all the content of your first seven energy bodies.

As you enter the mindstream through any of the five modes of Taoist meditation, you apply the inner dissolving process to release any and all bound shapes of energy that prevent the smooth flow of the mindstream. Along the way, you discover that you have an awareness both of the mind-stream and of those gaps where you become distracted and lose awareness of the mindstream. One of the primary jobs of the meditator is to fill in these gaps with an alive awareness, rather than numbing out or becoming distracted by panicking over a devastating piece of your mind's internal content. As you meditate and continuously release your deepest mental, emotional, psychic, and karmic tensions, you will sometimes enter into intermittent periods of stillness and emptiness, during which all your innermost tensions disappear. You then experience periods of peace and clarity that penetrate right to the core of your being.

These nurturing episodes come and go. Each interlude of stillness takes you to a more clear and relaxed inner location, from which you subsequently experience life. Each episode of stillness causes a deeper quieting of your internal world. After each bout of encountering emptiness, you will find yourself becoming ever more aware of the inner content and flow of the mindstream. Progressively, clarity comes from new qualities of your mindstream, relating to any of your first six energy bodies. By following and dissolving the content of your mindstream, your inner world eventually becomes completely still, empowering you then to become aware of Consciousness itself.

The Taoist Preparatory Practices: An Overview

CHAPTER
6

Lao Tse Tao Te Ching, Verse 76

Humans are born soft and flexible
In death they become stiff and hard
Plants are born soft and pliable
When dead they become brittle and dry

Therefore, those who are stiff and rigid
become disciples of death
While those who are soft and yielding
become disciples of life
The hard and stiff break
The soft and supple triumph

The Taoist Preparatory Practices: An Overview

All the basic practices of Taoism are geared toward developing practitioners into what Taoists call "complete human beings." In that state you are physically healthy, with energy flowing freely through unimpeded channels, and are ready for the rigors of more advanced practices. It is critical to master the preparatory work because, later on, when the spirit begins to open and you start converting Chi into spirit, the process can quite literally shock, agitate, or burn out an unprepared nervous system. Commonly, people's bodies cannot handle what occurs in the meditative spiritualization process, especially if fire methods are used. When the body's circuits reach a certain overloaded level, the mind/body can become ill.

To avoid such disintegration, you need to master the basic exercises for developing the downward currents of energy and for balancing the body's energy channels. (Remember, there are other directions for energy currents but only the downward direction is dealt with in this book for reasons of safety.) If you have been performing the breathing lessons in the Focus on Practice boxes, you have already started to learn one preparatory practice. In the preceding chapter you learned the fundamental techniques of Taoist standing meditation.

The preparatory practices are basic awareness exercises. Their purpose is to bring to conscious awareness all the essential energy flows in the body. (These flows are not, as many people think, solely the acupuncture meridian lines, although you can focus awareness on these also, if you so choose. The fire tradition emphasizes the acupuncture meridians more than the water tradition does.) In the initial part of the preparatory practices, you start to cleanse the physical body of any clogged energy inside of it. This process is undertaken to guide your mind to a point where it can communicate directly with the physical energy of your body. As an example, you should learn to be able to put your mind inside your liver to make it start secreting. Before you can accomplish this feat, you must learn to place your mind in your liver, to make it physically move, or at least have an awareness of what is happening there.

There are numerous energy lines in the body that are connected directly to your Consciousness.* These have a significant effect on how you think, how your body functions, how your spirit works, and how your psychic capacities emerge.

It is best to learn the energetic basics of chi gung prior to the more advanced practices of meditation, because such practices presume that you have the whole of the physical and chi bodies functioning as one completely integrated internal unit.** Your whole body should literally breathe and move as one cell. Everything—your muscles, ligaments, joints, internal organs, glands, brain centers, and the fluid around the spinal cord inside your spine—should literally be under the direct influence of (and moved by) your conscious ability as meditator. When the Taoists join the Consciousness and the thinking mind into one integrated, aware whole, they do it through the body. Unless the body energies are integrated and fully alive, it is difficult, if not impossible, to alchemically transmute the body's tissues in a fashion that unites with the Consciousness.

---

*For example, specific energy lines that run from the liver to the belly, heart, and brain explicitly regulate—for good or for ill—your physical body, emotions, and rational conceptions.

**See "The Sixteen-Part Nei Gung System" in Chapter 2.

It is also important that you develop the capacity to start moving your internal chi in synchronization with the natural pulsations of the energy of the earth (that is, the energies of the five elements; see Chapter 3) and of the cosmos— stars, planets, and satellite bodies such as our moon, asteroids, and comets, all of which naturally radiate energy that greatly influences the human body.

The first part of Taoist meditation practice, then, involves gaining total control of both your physical body and the chi that fuels the functioning of the human body, an achievement that forms the necessary infrastructure from which to start the intermediate practices of inner dissolving. Again, it is extremely important to learn chi gung first. These chi infrastructure practices are sometimes taught in unmoving seated postures, but mostly they are not. More commonly, they are taught through such Taoist arts as tai chi, ba gua, the other internal martial arts, chi gung, basic standing postures, Taoist yoga, and sexual chi gung.

To label normal standing or moving chi gung as "meditation" is, to a certain degree, misrepresentation, as these practices have no consequential effect on the deeper layers of your consciousness.* They do, however, prepare you for meditation and moreover have many external physical, chi, and emotional benefits. For example, at the basic level of calming the agitated mind, they can be very effective. Generally speaking, in the beginning, moving and standing chi gung, tai chi, ba gua, sexual chi gung, and Taoist yoga are better for your external health than are the inner dissolving practices done sitting. Each of these methods develops your physical strength and overall health. They also increase the ability of your central nervous system to handle the stresses

---

*Tai chi, ba gua, and chi gung methods that come from the Chinese martial arts and medical communities (which comprise almost all of what is available in the West) are *not* meditation. They are, however, meditative in nature. Taoism has ways of doing tai chi that function as meditation in that they are specifically constructed to free human Consciousness completely. Although both methods may appear to have similar motions when looked at externally, in actuality the Taoist meditation methods use internal consciousness work normally absent in the martial arts and medical chi traditions.

and challenges of day-to-day living in a breathlessly fast, computer-driven era.

The sitting mode is generally reserved for more advanced intermediate and concluding-stage practices. In these later stages, the sitting mode is more efficient for exploring the most internal aspects of your consciousness. In Taoism, you need good sitting practices, by means of which the ultimate goals of internal alchemy and meditation can be realized.

Preparatory chi practices are easy to learn. In summary, their purpose is dual: (a) to calm the distracted mind so that your consciousness does not jump around disconnected from your core like a frightened rabbit, and (b) to open up the energy channels of the body to make you physically strong and energetically stable. When you sit for a prolonged time, if your body is strong, the effects of gravity do not distract your mind. The last thing a meditating mind needs is distraction, which gravity can bring regardless of whatever position you meditate in. When your channels are open and energetically stable, you can release the muck-and-grime dysfunctional blockages encrusting your Consciousness in a much smoother and less shocking way to the central nervous system than if your channels were closed. This avoids physical problems and emotional or psychic "freakouts."

A Word about Taoist Yoga

Taoist yoga can also be of great value in forming a foundation for more advanced meditation practices. Taoist yoga is somewhat akin to a more simplified hatha yoga, but the focus in Taoist yoga is on what happens to the chi and body systems internally, beneath the skin, rather than on large external muscular stretching movements. In Taoist yoga the external movement of the body and the postures are created by *specifically using the internal components of chi gung methodology* to move chi in the body and to release energy blockage in the physical tissues. By moving the body in this fashion, the chi in the organs, glands, and spine is directly engaged, whereas the muscles primarily are involved in a large external stretch. In Taoist yoga the breath is always continuous and circular, in contrast to the holding of the breath in hatha and Tibetan yoga.* As a matter of fact, most of the stretches in Taoist yoga tend not to be nearly as extreme as those of Hatha yoga. The latter usually concentrates on sheer muscular stretching, rather than on the Taoist yoga approach of internally releasing the insides to create external movement, a totally different process. Yet these great yoga traditions are more similar than they are different.

FOCUS ON PRACTICE
Taoist Internal Breathing, Lesson 9

When you begin, it is natural to first fill up the front of the body and next progress to the sides. After a while, however, it is best if you can expand and relax the front and sides of your belly and return to your originating center line *simultaneously and not sequentially.*

---

*Circular breathing means that there is no stopping of the breathing cycle—no holding of the breath occurs either in inhalation or exhalation.

THE WAY OF LIU
The Story of Hui Neng

 My teacher Liu learned the foundation practices of Taoism through the Taoist internal martial arts tradition of China. He then became recognized as enlightened in the Mahayana Tien Tai school of Chinese Buddhism and only afterward, in the mountains of western China, learned the subtleties of Taoist internal alchemy. I told Liu that I had studied Zen Buddhism since my teens and then asked him about the internal structure of studying Consciousness and meditation in Taoism. He replied by telling the story of Hui Neng, one of the major patriarchs in Chan (Zen) Buddhism.*

When Hui Neng entered the monastery, he was asked not so much to sit and meditate but rather to work in food production, to make himself useful in the normal daily routine of his fellow residents. First he spent time laboring in the rice fields and drying the rice, which strengthened his body. After doing this work for a while he moved into the grinding room, where he applied the same grinding action day after day with a pestle to separate the rice kernel from its husk. In the mornings and evenings he would sit for a short time and meditate, but mostly he would grind the rice for ten hours a day. Initially, with each monotonous circling of the grinding stone, he would become involved with grinding the rice "the right or the best way." As time passed, he would begin to focus less on the action of grinding (at which he was becoming progressively more efficient) and more on observing the workings of his mind and chi as the wheel turned and turned. In his morning and afternoon meditations, he began to learn sitting chi gung, the inner Chi work of Chan Buddhism.

*Chan Buddhism was created in central China from the marriage of Taoism and Buddhism during the sixth century A.D. The health and spiritual aspects of the Taoist inner Chi work were seamlessly integrated into Chan's basic sitting meditation methods. When Chan moved to Japan, it was renamed Zen. Although the spiritual and philosophical aspects of Chan Buddhism were imported to Japan, Chan's chi practices derived from Taoism were not. Generally speaking, Chan Buddhism has a softer and less military bent than its Japanese or Korean versions.

THE WAY OF LIU
The Story of Hui Neng (continued)

As more time wore on, Hui Neng became aware of how the subtle thoughts and emotions (frustration, greed, hate, lust, sloth, viciousness, jealousy, hope, fear, anger, despair, and all kinds of desires) arose as he ground away at the rice. Slowly he found himself projecting all of his emotions into the rice as he became attached to the grain, handled it, became lethargic toward it, frustrated with it, and fell in and out of love with it. In each grain of rice he slowly began to see the past, present, and future merge into one, and still he ground on, until all of his deepest subliminal thoughts surfaced and spoke through the rice. He gradually became aware of his spirit as his thoughts and psychic sensations were ground into Consciousness without content. As he ground away, emptiness began to appear spontaneously in his mind. Slowly, Hui Neng's mind/consciousness became completely empty and still. Each turn of the wheel produced life-giving rice and at the same time freed his being to be at peace with itself.

He ground on, hour after hour, millions of times, until the rice was the rice and his Consciousness was his Consciousness, each in its natural place, neither confused nor commingled.

The millions of grindings of rice simply took away from Hui Neng all that was not intrinsically his self. He was left with his pure unbound Consciousness. The grinding of the rice was simply a tool, a medium to practice on. It was the clearing of Hui's consciousness that was the primary benefit from the point of view of meditation. The by-product of ground rice for sustaining the body was a wise way of killing two birds with one stone.

Liu then explained how the five modes of training for the preparatory chi practices are actually the physical media through which virtually all human activities take place. These five practices are in effect the same as the activity of grinding the rice. Initially, they make the body healthy and strong. Then they develop the mind's ability to dispassionately observe its various mind/body/spirit interactions and connections, or lack thereof. Later, the emotional maturity/stillness techniques release the bindings of the emotional and mental bodies, allowing the individual to become free of undue influence by the past and thus setting the stage for emotional maturity.

Ultimately, each sitting session or chi gung or tai chi set or Taoist sexual encounter further refines the consciousness. The normal consciousness is led further and further into emptiness

THE WAY OF LIU
The Story of Hui Neng (continued)

and eventually stillness, all the while enabling the practitioner to maintain the strength and vigor of youth when standing, moving, sitting, lying, or having sexual relations. The five modes of practice, like the lifting and grinding of the rice, simply become a way to refine one's consciousness, one's method of meditation. In truth, the modes of Taoist Chi practices are, like the growing, drying, lifting, and grinding of rice, only the media that emphasize different aspects of life; they are not the art of meditation itself.

The Moving Mode of Taoist Practice

Taoist tradition contains many moving meditation forms. Some use only a few simple movements, while others, such as tai chi and ba gua, comprise a complex series of movements. All begin as health-oriented chi gung preparatory practices and later lead to the same inner enlightenment that is the goal of the sitting and sexual meditation practices—on the road to becoming one with the Tao.

Moving meditation practices are more difficult to execute than the standing practice described in Chapter 5. They require you not only to stay aware of your mindstream but also to maintain everything you did while standing, *plus* cultivate balanced, integrated external movement, *plus* add an emotional dimension. The movements can and do cause deep internal shifting that can potentially activate the repressed emotions stored in our physical tissue.

When you undergo powerful emotional experiences, expressed or repressed, your body usually stores them in some sort of external or internal vibratory "shape" fashioned by pressures and tensions below the skin. Most beginning practitioners of moving meditation move only their surface muscles in much the same way the muscles normally move during calisthenics. But chi gung, tai chi, and ba gua were designed so that their physical twistings—the motion they evoke in the fascia, ligaments, joints, and internal organs—progressively penetrate the body, causing deep internal pressures. These pressures bring about superior health and ameliorate diseases. One of the reasons these internal pressures benefit health is that often, over time, unresolved or suppressed emotions embedded in your body can cause both pain and physical malfunction. The moving practices release those embedded emotions, thereby fixing the physical malfunctions they cause. In fact, the moving practices give you better access to those stuck emotions and a more effective way of releasing them than the standing practice does.

One difficulty to overcome, though, is that in the early phases of learning moving practices, a large part of your effort goes into attending to all the details involved in learning external physical movements, making it hard to focus totally on the mindstream itself. For that reason moving meditation practices begin with an emphasis on how to perform the physical movements, with increasing attention to the specific body sensations you want to activate and how, when, and where you want to move energy inside your body. With the skills learned in standing meditation, you then begin to recognize and feel the subliminally stored tension (energy shapes) in your body and discover a way to release that tension while moving your body. Then you may begin the process of quieting the mind and following the mindstream.

Moving Meditation with Feet Fixed in Place, Body Moving

First Movement of Tai Chi for Meditation (Wu Style Tai Chi)

The purpose of this moving meditation is, with physical motion, to give you a sense of energy moving through your body and a sense of the dissolving process while you are moving. First try to achieve the internal body alignments introduced in the standing meditation exercise described in Chapter 5 in order to create a proper body posture that does not waste, block, or dissipate chi. In doing this exercise, please remember these important points about your knees: (1) your kneecaps are never to extend past your toes, and (2) when bending or straightening, keep your kneecaps still and move your buttocks up and down instead. If you find bending and straightening your knees from your buttocks to be difficult, forget the instructions about bending and straightening the knees and concentrate only on the instructions for the arms.

Just as in the standing meditation exercise you spent about a week at each level (relaxing just the head, then the head and chest, then the head, chest, and belly, etc.), you likewise should plan to spend sufficient time mastering each of the following steps before progressing on to the next one. Be patient, and expect the entire process to take several weeks.

Step 1. The Physical Movement

(1a)   Stand with your feet parallel, approximately shoulder width apart. Open up the underside of your pelvis so that your shins are parallel. Do not collapse your knees inward or stand bowlegged in any way. Relax your pelvis and tuck it forward so your tailbone faces downward, rather than backward. Keep your back and neck straight, with your head lightly lifted, leaning neither forward, back, nor to either side. Allow your shoulders to become heavy until they feel like they are sinking down to your hips. Keep your armpits slightly open in order to avoid blocking the energy flowing through your left and right channels. Throughout step 1, do your best to prevent having your shoulders raise up into the air. During all of the following arm and hand movements, neither your hands nor arms should come closer than the distance of a fist to your body. This principle will enhance your chi flow. Your hands are at your sides, palms facing backward.

(1b)   Now focus your mind on relaxing your whole body, especially your shoulders, elbows, wrists, and hands. Gently encourage your mind to travel inside your body down from your shoulders to your elbows and fingertips, keeping your elbows slightly bent. In a circular, arcing motion, slowly raise your wrists upward and forward in the air to shoulder height. Let your wrists bend and relax, and gently allow your fingers and elbow tips to point toward the ground. Through numerous repetitions let your wrists and elbows become parallel to each other, slightly less than the width of your shoulders, in line with your left and right channels. As your hands rise up in the air, simultaneously bend your knees and elbows 20–30 percent (initially no more than two to four inches). To both bend and straighten your knees *do not* move your kneecaps forward, backward, or sideways. Rather, keeping your kneecaps still, raise and lower your buttocks to bend or straighten the backs of your knees only a few inches.

(1c)   When your hands reach shoulder height, simultaneously shift your weight forward to the balls of your feet, straighten your knees and elbows slightly, and very slightly straighten your wrists and extend your fingers straight ahead of you. In extending your arms, it is important that you do not fully straighten your elbows; doing so will block the relaxed circulation of your chi.

(1d)   Now simultaneously shift your weight back to the center of your feet and slowly pull your hands and elbows back toward your shoulders. Your elbows comfortably move to the back of your body as you bend your knees slightly. Your elbow tips will gradually move further backward and go slightly behind your sides, as your wrists bend and your hands come back to the front of your shoulders. Then let your elbows and palms push toward the floor, coming to rest on the sides of your body. As you shift your weight back onto your heels, your wrists bend further. Now push your palms down (feel as if you are pushing water down your body to below your feet). Simultaneously, your elbows and knees straighten to about 80 percent of their potential extension. Your palms finish at your sides, facing downward. Do not lock either your elbows or knees. You have now completed the movement.

(1e)　From here, just repeat 1b to 1d over and over again. Move slowly, but not so slowly that you easily become distracted. Find the speed at which you can best be continuously aware of your body alignments and body movements, without spacing out or losing the flow of awareness. After you can do this four-part motion, move at whatever slow speed you find where you can best relax every part of your body, keeping your attention continuous, without becoming fixated or distracted. If you do find your mind drifting, just go back to the beginning of the movement and start afresh. After you can do this complete motion for *five to ten minutes without stopping*, your relaxed concentration will have grown significantly, and it is time for step 2. Again, if you find bending and straightening your knees from your buttocks to be difficult for you, forget the instructions for the legs and concentrate only on the instructions for the arms.

Step 2. Relax and Release

(2a)　Next become aware of how your body feels. Where does it feel tense or tight? In the beginning, pay special attention to your neck, shoulders, and belly. As you move your body, progressively relax your muscles. Gradually, you will be able to feel the inside of your body with more confidence. You will begin to feel all sorts of things inside your body below your surface muscles.

(2b)   When you do this motion and relax deeper inside your muscles toward the bone, you will find yourself being able to stretch your muscles by simply releasing the tension and strength inside them rather than actively forcing or pushing to stretch them out.

(2c)   In the beginning, your arms and shoulders will begin to unwind and stretch. Keep your spine straight and do not slump. Keep your eyes straight ahead without tilting your head in any direction. In stages, the stretching will extend to your back, legs, and then your belly.

(2d)   Gradually release all your strength, until you feel it dropping out of your upper body, then to your belly, and then to your legs and feet. As you do this, your feet will feel more rooted in the earth, and your mind will become calmer and calmer.

(2e)   There may be a tendency to lose your continuous awareness when you deeply relax a particular body part or after you release and stretch a particular muscle or joint. It will again be important not to space out. If you do, begin again without self-recrimination. After you can do this initial tai chi motion for *five to ten minutes without stopping*, your relaxed concentration will have grown significantly and it is time for step 3.

Step 3. Consciously Move Energy within Your Body

A dimension of energy movement is now added to the actual physical movement. If you cannot yet feel energy moving in your body, imagine it moving as indicated.

(3a)   As your wrists rise to your shoulders, pull the flow of energy from below your feet, up through your body to above your head. Coordinate your rising hands and the energy movement so that when your hands go higher, your energy moves higher.

(3b)   Coordinate the extending of your wrist and fingers forward with letting the energy project out of your fingers into space. In the beginning, project energy only a short distance and within your limits, so you do not create internal strain by trying to do more than you are yet able to. With practice, you will become able to effortlessly project your energy, farther and farther away from you. If you cannot actually feel energy yet, simply imagine it occurring and stay focused on your intent.

(3c)   As your hands withdraw to just in front of your chest, simultaneously let the energy that you have just projected away from you flow back through space and into your fingers. Next, let it flow progressively into your hand, wrists, elbows, and then to your shoulders and spine and heart.

(3d)   As your palms move down your sides, simultaneously encourage your energy to flow down your body. When you feel the energy move of its own accord, guide it gently with your mind, first to your belly, then your legs, and finally to your feet and below the ground.

After you are satisfied that you can do step 3 for *five to ten minutes without stopping*, your relaxed concentration will have grown significantly, and it is time for step 4.

Step 4. Put Your Mind in Your Tantien

(4a)   You now want to allow some part of your mind's awareness to drop down from your brain into your belly. Keep this up until you experience the sensation (which progressively grows from vague to distinct) of thinking from your lower tantien rather than your head.

(4b)   Next, focus on gradually being aware of your internal energies spreading from your lower tantien in ever-larger circles, until your belly gains the ability to feel every part of your body simultaneously. So if some part of your body feels right or wrong, you gain this knowledge from your gut, which feels without doubt what is happening in your body. You do not gain it from your talking head, which analyzes if *maybe* this or that *could* be happening to your body.

After you are satisfied that you can do step 4 for *five to ten minutes without stopping*, your relaxed concentration will have grown significantly.

FOCUS ON A SPECIAL TOPIC
From Movement Comes Stillness, and from Stillness Comes Movement: The Relationship between Chi and Emptiness

 Body energy produces Chi energy, which in turn produces spirit and the opening of the heart/mind, which in turn produces emptiness and internal stillness. In whichever of the five practice modalities a meditator chooses to use, after he or she has arrived at emptiness and stillness and continues to practice, *the process reverses* and the circle completes itself, presuming that the practitioner's energy channels have been properly prepared.

When applied to moving meditation, this process produces the standard Taoist dictum: From movement of body and Chi comes stillness/emptiness, and from stillness/emptiness comes spirit and movement of Chi and body. If, when in the sitting mode, one goes deeply to stillness and stabilizes there and continues to practice sitting, chi energy will begin to accumulate in the lower tantien, then spill over, flooding and nourishing the energy channels of the body, healing illness,

FOCUS ON A SPECIAL TOPIC
From Movement Comes Stillness, and from Stillness Comes Movement: The Relationship between Chi and Emptiness
(continued)

and greatly strengthening the body.* This experience is normally strongly felt in the hands and fingers, just as happens in chi gung when a tremendous amount of energy is being generated. This "creation of internal power" derived from sitting was part of the historical reason internal martial artists practiced sitting meditation, even if they had no interest in spirituality per se.

Therefore, in any Taoist meditation mode, there is great benefit to continuing to practice after one initially enters into any level of stillness. Tai chi and ba gua are both well known and respected as great moving meditation methods because one of the primary prerequisites for practicing these arts at an advanced level is maintaining a still, empty mind. As the stillness deepens, it simultaneously causes the chi to concentrate in the lower tantien and then to spill over and energize the whole body.

Moving, Balance, and Meditation

We now extend our moving meditation to becoming aware of balance, that much-needed commodity in our increasingly unnatural world. You encounter balance each time you lift your foot in the air and put it down.

Lift your foot, put it down, and shift your weight to your other foot, left-right-left-right. There is no need to lift your foot more than a few inches, although you can lift it

---

*How to open the energy channels constituted a portion of the methods taught by the Taoists to the original Chan (Zen) practitioners in China. Unfortunately, when Chan was imported to Japan, these methods did not transfer with it. These methods, included within the Taoist nei gung system (see Chapter 2), can greatly benefit the health of meditators, whatever their school or doctrine, who engage in quiet sitting and are able to enter into emptiness.

higher if you so desire. By constantly lifting your foot and shifting your weight, you gain insight into how your mind and body can become more balanced. By being very attentive to the details of maintaining your physical balance, you can slowly begin to see how the balance between your emotional and intellectual thoughts shift between turning inward or outward, or thinking or feeling this way or that, in terms of whatever energy occurs. Through persistent practice, the swirling polarities begin to come into balanced perspective and settle down. When your mind becomes still, you begin to see the place in your mind that generates both polarities but is neither.* This insight, over time, allows you to comprehend the nature of change itself.

A journey of a thousand miles begins with one step. In the West, most people are fairly aware of their upper bodies but not so aware of their legs and feet. Most Westerners can feel every tiny part of their hands easily but are not equally sensitive to their feet, which is what we use to walk. Initially, then, we must become aware of our feet.

Once again, be sure to take the necessary time to become fully confident with each step before progressing to the next one.

Step 1

(1a)   Stand with both feet separated, no wider than hip width apart. Be aware of your physical balance. With your weight on your right leg, begin to easily pick your left foot up, at least to ankle height, and put it down. Do the same with your right foot. Alternate, left-right-left, and so on.

(1b)   Stand still again and begin to let your mind feel your legs, ultimately ending with feeling every part of your foot. After you can get a solid sensation of your foot, begin (with your weight on your right foot) to lift your left foot up in the air and put

---

*In Chinese philosophical thought, this concept is termed *tai chi*, from which the martial art tai chi chuan derives its name.

it back down four or five times, all the while keeping awareness of your moving foot and not losing it. Repeat this action with your right foot, until your awareness is continuously focused on your moving foot. The moving foot will be the focus of your awareness in all of the exercises in this section.

When we walk, most of us are preoccupied with where we are headed and not with what is happening deep inside our bodies as we move along. This lack of inner awareness causes us to lose much of the joy of life.

(1c) Now do some silent marching up and down, giving more energy to everything you did in (1a) and (1b). This activity will be quite helpful for older people or for those with lower-body injuries who have a greater than average tendency to disconnect mentally from their feet.

Step 2

We now increase the foot awareness exercise to include awareness of nonphysical energy. Bring one foot up to comfortably touch the ankle, shin, or knee of your other leg. This simple move, repeated, will gradually increase your balance. Do this for a while until your balance stabilizes.

(2a) Be aware of the difference in feeling when your foot is touching the ground and when it is off the ground.

(2b) Be aware of or at least in the beginning have the idea of how you can let the earth's energy flow up into your foot from the ground when you raise your foot.

(2c) Be aware of how you can let energy drop down from your foot into the earth as your foot comes down and touches the ground.

(2d) Let your awareness start at your tailbone and over

time move deeper and deeper into and through your leg, until the awareness and physical and energetic sensations reach and put pressure on three points on the sole of your foot: the ball of your foot, the heel, and the center of the arch. Become aware of the energies each naturally generates inside your body. Putting pressure on the ball of the foot (the "bubbling well" acupuncture point) causes energy to rise up the body. Putting pressure on the heel point causes energy to sink down the body. Working with pressure on the foot's arch allows you to balance the rising and falling currents.

Step 3

(3a)   Continuing to stay aware of the bottom of your foot, pick up your foot a few inches and kick it forward gently, straight in front of you. Begin with the foot fairly stiff and gradually relax the ankle completely, letting it flop as you gently kick your foot. The looser the ankle becomes, the faster it flops, and the more attention will be required to stay focused on the ankle, sole, and toes of the foot in a mentally relaxed manner. Alternate left and right feet, and kick five or six times.

(3b)   In this stage, you will still gently kick your foot, only you let it cross your body (right foot to left side and vice versa), in the manner of an old-time vaudeville dancer. After five or six kicks of both legs, your mind should have acquired the ability to remain conscious of both feet while moving them, and your balance should have increased significantly.

Step 4

Now let's focus attention on both mental and physical balance. Shift your weight side to side, bringing one leg up to touch the other leg (somewhere comfortably from ankle to your knee) after you have finished the weight shift. As you move from the left to the right foot, pay attention to any idea or concept that naturally comes to mind. As you shift your weight, focus on the opposite side of the concept—what you want and don't want, why it's good or bad, high or low, tasteful or obnoxious, smart or stupid, correct or incorrect, and so on. When you are on one leg, completely focus mentally on one side of the concept; on the other leg, take the opposite position. Side to side, side to side, strive to keep your physical and mental balance until in the middle a quiet, still space begins to appear and you are able, in a relaxed fashion, to see both opposites existing simultaneously in your awareness. Here you can naturally enter the mindstream, or at the very least a strong meditative state.

    (4a)   Stand with both feet shoulder width apart. Next keep your awareness simultaneously *on both feet* throughout the whole exercise. Shift your weight completely onto your right foot. Concentrate on the motion as your left thigh first shifts over to the right, immediately followed by your left foot, which lifts off the ground to touch your ankle, calf, or knee. Pause for a second or two, continuing to be aware of the soles of both feet.

    (4b)   With your weight on your right foot, stretch and extend your left foot sideways to the left several inches past where it previously had been placed and let it touch the ground. Next, let your hip and belly start shifting sideways toward the left. Then let your right foot leave the ground as your right thigh moves toward your left thigh. Finally, with all your weight on your left leg, let your right foot touch your left ankle, calf, or knee.

    (4c)   Now repeat 4b, 4a, 4b, 4a, shifting right-left-right-left, and so on, for as long as you can, each time moving ever deeper into the mindstream.

How to Stay in the Mindstream While You Are Moving

First, the movements of your chosen moving meditation form must be practiced sufficiently to have become second nature, so you can remember and do the sequence of movements without any strain. The simpler and fewer in number the individual movements are, the easier the task. The longer and more complex movement patterns—such as tai chi, whose forms have anywhere from 16 to 128 movements—will need to be practiced until they are absolutely hardwired into your muscle memory, so that you do not have to struggle to retrieve them. You know that it is in your muscle memory when, if you have a movement hiccup and miss a beat, you consciously pick up the thread of the lost movement again without experiencing anxiety, panic, or confusion that arises from feeling lost.

Second, your breathing must be sufficiently smooth so you can notice any micro-variations in it. These subtle changes are cues that help you become aware that something is happening subliminally inside of you, which you will want to bring into your conscious awareness.

Third, your energy should be strong enough while doing the form that you can stay fully mentally present in your body more often than spacing out. This prerequisite ability is one that a Taoist mediation practitioner would normally acquire while learning to do standing chi gung. By this juncture, the energy of your lower tantien should be stable enough to act as an anchor for your awareness. Eventually, you want to be completely present during the whole practice, both in your awareness in general and in your lower tantien in particular. At this point, you should be confident that your physical and chi bodies are stable. A competent teacher can verify this for you.

Fourth, as your arms, legs, and body execute movements in space, you must become aware of the emotional, mental, psychic, and causal sensations that are naturally continuously arising, changing, and moving within both your physical body and mind. The ability to feel ever more subtle internal sensations can come only from long hours of practice; it never comes from intellectual pondering alone. Any agitated sensations will first need to be dissolved to reduce the gross mental noise that will distract you from the more subtle mindstream. After some indeterminate time (less for some, more for others) and prolonged struggle with dissolving the grosser blockages, the mind, in stages, will begin to gain the strength to be aware of the mindstream itself.

Fifth, the mindstream can be very subtle. It is like a golden thread that runs through all your awareness, just on the razor's edge of the conscious and unconscious parts of yourself. This subtle but powerful mind thread connects all your energies to consciousness itself. It will first appear to be moving all around the body and playing hide-and-seek with your awareness. When you first contact the mindstream, do not attempt to dissolve its contents. For now, simply do your best to stay with the mindstream. Feel it and become aware of all the nuances that are part of it. In time, you will be able to stay with the mindstream for an entire set of tai chi or ba gua or chi gung.

Sixth, although you may first recognize the mindstream as appearing to be inside your body, it is actually a function of Consciousness itself and therefore simultaneously exists within your whole physical body and outside it in space. To focus on all of this at once would be a needlessly overwhelming task. There is, however, a shortcut.

The lower, middle, and upper tantiens (see p. 104) all lie on the central energy channel. Any of these three is a direct connection to the mindstream and, eventually, Universal Consciousness itself. The mindstream can be continuously observed and accessed from any of the three. Each of the three tantiens are like a riverbed, upon which you can watch the river's water (the mindstream) flowing. Floating in that water will be all sorts of twigs and leaves (the content of your first six energy bodies). You now want to dissolve any perceived content you encounter, without leaving the mindstream. The procedure: stay focused on only a single tantien during a complete moving practice, and from that one tantien only, stay in contact with the mindstream. After you can be aware of the mindstream without major gaps for three sets of movements in a row, then progress forward to dissolving whatever internal content is commingled with the mindstream in your awareness.

In order to kill two birds with one stone, most meditators usually begin with the lower tantien. This way of proceeding strengthens the body's ability to withstand whatever emotional or physical shocks are released from the energy of the mindstream's internal content.

If you wish to deal with the psychic side of your nature, lack of mental clarity, or compulsive emotions, focus the procedure on your upper tantien, inside your brain. If you wish to sort out what the nature of relationship to other sentient beings is in all its shades and hues, then focus on the middle tantien, at your heart.

The classic Taoist water-method strategy for entering into the seventh body (the body of individuality) is first, to work with the lower tantien, then to work with the upper tantien. Next, the energies from each of these tantiens is moved to the heart. Here, you relax into your being, discovering and stabilizing Universal Consciousness until your heart center is alive with the living presence of its light.

Summary

On the road taken to relaxing into your being, your personal practice and effort will gradually reveal phenomena to your conscious mind, in this order: (1) awareness of the subtle physical and energetic sensations of your body; (2) an awareness of awareness itself; (3) an awareness of the mindstream itself; (4) the energetic internal residue content of your first six energy bodies embedded in the mindstream; and (5) the universal nature of Consciousness itself. Each of these five stages is different, and each is realized through practice (and never through mere theorizing). Each in turn allows you to relax more deeply into the core of your being and, eventually, completely relax into the Universal Consciousness itself.

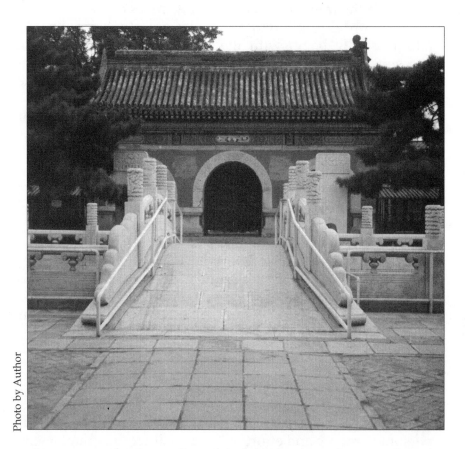

Gateway to the Inner Temple of the Bai Yun Guan in Beijing. The author spent many hours here practicing the Taoist meditation techniques he learned from Liu Hung Chieh.

The Intermediate Stage of Practice: Meditation and Stillness

CHAPTER
7

I Ching : Hexagram 15–Humility

Ghosts and demons harm the complacent
And raise up the humble

The Intermediate Stage of Practice: Meditation and Stillness

The Road to Emotional Maturity

After sufficient time with preparatory practices, one moves into the next stage of Taoist meditation, which initially involves a subject of great interest to everyone in the Western world: emotion. The Western world, especially America, tends to be fascinated by emotional issues. Witness the huge industries—from the entertainment media to psychotherapy—that thrive on dealing with and manipulating emotions.

From the preparatory practices you will have developed some understanding of both the physical and the chi bodies. In the intermediate or middle stage you start to pinpoint where the emotional blockages are, inside both the chi body and the physical body, and you discover the emotions corresponding to these blocks. You then use a variety of practices, mostly based on the inner dissolving process, to go through what the Chinese call "dealing with your ghosts." These "ghosts" consist of all your memories and everything else that is not present at the moment but nonetheless can strongly affect you. Everyone carries within himself or herself the baggage of jangled emotional patterns. People can harbor emotional blockages that were formed in childhood or even, in fact, in the womb.

Intermediate (Middle) Practices

The aim of the middle practices is to attain inner stillness and to become aware of Universal Consciousness. The benefits of the middle practices include gaining emotional harmony and releasing structural blockages in your emotions, including traumas and fixations.

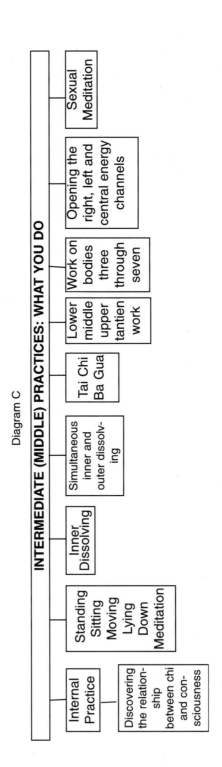

Diagram C

Pre-Birth Considerations: Resolving Birth Traumas and Dissolving Blockages from DNA to Birth

In Buddhism, the birth trauma is one of the four causes of suffering (the others are old age, sickness, and death). Birth traumas can be immensely destabilizing for people.* Emotional patterns from addictions to anger to depression may be locked into a person's psychological makeup from birth. A person may be born a fighter owing to the genuine struggle that occurred when he or she went through the extensive hours of a difficult delivery. Fighting one's way through the birth channel can certainly shape behavior for life. So can being pulled forcefully into the world, as may be the case with a baby who has literally given up in the womb. An infant undergoing a birth like this may experience depression for the rest of its life. Any number of different events can happen to a person at birth or while in the womb. Whatever they are, such episodes or ordeals can be dealt with effectively through the inner dissolving practices.

Behavior patterns resulting from birth traumas are frozen in place by energy blocks. By dissolving these blocks, you can make these patterns vanish for good. However, this process succeeds fully only if the dissolving practice is taken to virtual completion.

In the intermediate stage of Taoist meditation, you become significantly more conscious of various energies that are not really what we ordinarily feel as "physical." However, these energies are a part of your body. As your body cultivates increased Chi, it becomes progressively more important to be extremely aware. There is a mind-body-energy interaction that is undeniable. Within your body's energy are stored memories of what you have undergone from the day you were conceived. Through Taoist meditation, we tap into this cellular memory. Taoism, as well as the esoteric traditions of Buddhism and, to a certain extent, some schools of

---

*Such traumas include a variety of physical situations that can strongly imprint an infant's central nervous system: the umbilical cord being wrapped around the baby's neck, breech birth, the skull being dented by forceps, etc.

modern psychology, holds that the body retains memories from the womb, even from the time you were a DNA code.

Those pre-birth memories are conditionings. Commonly, they do not allow a person to become mature, because they constantly throw one back to the past. The dissolving techniques are used to "dissolve" the whole of the body, inch by inch, until every blockage that is inside a body is dispersed. The water method of Taoism strongly applies this dissolving, or the breaking up of energy, in the same way that water wears away a rock. It is similar to placing sugar in water. After a while, the sugar dissolves and the water completely absorbs it. In like manner, through application of the Taoist meditative dissolving technique, emotional tensions and blockages disappear.

FOCUS ON A SPECIAL TOPIC
Can Taoist Meditation
Replace Psychotherapy?

 A question frequently raised is, Can the dissolving practices of Taoist meditation completely replace the need for psychiatric care? The answer for deeply troubled, emotionally unstable, and psychologically dysfunctional people is no. However, seeing a psychotherapist does not automatically preclude becoming involved with Taoist meditation. Many undergo psychotherapy for support, not for treatment of severe mental aberrations for which hospitalization or out-patient psychiatric care is required. Those tending toward mental instability, though, may not be able to handle meditation. In modern life, nearly all of us have to earn a living and interact with others. It is extremely difficult to withdraw for extended periods to the sanctuary of a monastery or ashram where all needs are taken care of while one's severe personal problems are worked through. Psychotherapy is much more appropriate for dealing with the dysfunctions that derive from a level of emotional development where someone is incapable of taking responsibility for his or her own emotions or behavior.

FOCUS ON PRACTICE
Taoist Internal Breathing, Lesson 10:
Lower Back Breathing

- Concentrate on the inhale, expanding from your center line to your spine and backward to your skin, lower back muscles, and all the way up and into your kidneys. Return to your original position on the exhale.
- Breathing from your kidneys will be harder than breathing from your front and sides. Initially, it helps to lie down on the floor, knees up in the air, soles of the feet on the floor, with the lower part of your back firmly pressing the floor. The pressure of your body pressing into the floor on the inhale, and the release of the pressure on the exhale, will make it easier to feel the inside of your body.

Breathing with the kidneys is considered very important in Taoist practices. In traditional Chinese medicine, the kidneys are held to be the source of a human's overall vitality and sexual/procreative capacity. Energizing the kidneys is of particularly significant importance in terms of developing a healthy body and clear mind. Chronic exhaustion often reflects weakness in the kidneys.

- Progress from two breaths to twenty, with continuous awareness.
- Now build from twenty to thirty breaths, using all parts of your abdominal cavity simultaneously (rather than sequentially). On the inhale, expand from the center line of your belly to the front, side, and back (kidneys). Return to your original position on the exhale.
- On the inhale, expand your belly like a tube, from its center line, between the solar plexus and the lower tantien, simultaneously forward, backward, and sideways. Return your belly to its original position on the exhale.
- On the inhale, your belly should simultaneously expand as you follow your breath from your nose to lower tantien. On your exhale, you should follow your breath back from your tantien, up the center line of your body, and out your nose, as you let your belly return to its original position.

FOCUS ON PRACTICE
Taoist Internal Breathing, Lesson 10:
Lower Back Breathing (continued)

This method of breathing will provide a wonderful massage for your internal organs. You can breath in this manner twenty-four hours a day once this new physical breathing method becomes a comfortable habit. Just as massaging your muscles adds to their tone and overall functioning, so will this breathing method benefit your internal organs. In terms of your health, massaging your internal organs is more important than toning your muscles. Just as muscle massage increases your overall blood circulation, this breathing increases the blood circulation in those deeper blood vessels that nourish the internal organs. This type of breathing may increase the mass of your stomach muscles and definitely will make them stronger.

Build from two to twenty and then to thirty breaths. Make sure you breathe to only 70 percent of your capacity. Do not expand your breath to more than is comfortable. You introduce an effortlessness into your breathing by both taking less air with each breath than you can, and simultaneously relaxing your nerves with each inhale and exhale. Regardless of how much time you take to complete one inhale and exhale (ten seconds to minutes), this effortlessness in the physical act of breathing is of tremendous benefit. It continuously reduces your stress as well as strengthens your internal organs, overall body vitality, and mental clarity.

Effortlessness is also critical in developing continuous awareness of your mindstream, without mental tension. Mental tension saps your mental and physical stamina and ability to concentrate continuously for long periods of time without becoming tired or distracted.

For severely disturbed people psychiatric care is more appropriate than Taoist meditation, and meditation cannot normally substitute for it. Taoist meditation was designed for those who can cope with day-to-day realities, both in the external world and inside themselves. Classically, people with severe mental disorders had to work through their crippling psychological problems before being accepted as meditation students. This is still true today.

Yet the majority of today's psychotherapy clients do not go for, nor do they need, treatment for severe mental aberrations. Rather, they go for a myriad of life-affirming reasons, including general support, marriage and family counseling, counseling in times of crisis—death, divorce, or rape—achieving high performance, learning more about their human potential, and so on. Much of today's psychotherapy is intended to help work past such normal emotional and psychic glitches, which almost everyone has, and which prevent the full flowing of Consciousness. For those without crippling psychiatric dysfunction, psychotherapy can be an excellent preparation for, and adjunct to, Taoist meditation. On the other side of the coin, for persons involved in psychotherapy, adding Taoist meditation practices can deepen the process, helping them to resolve their issues more quickly.

Taoists believe that humans can transform themselves. In classic Taoist meditation, worthy students recognize and understand that resolving their emotional problems is ultimately their own personal responsibility. Despite whatever might have been done to them, they do not hold others to be the ultimate cause of, or solution to their emotional problems. Taoists believe that only when students have reached such a state of mind can they use the dissolving techniques responsibly to resolve their inner conflicts, without blaming or attacking others as the source of their own misery and without inflicting pain or death (to themselves or anyone else) to get back at others.

When you start progressing through all the different ways of dissolving your emotions (which naturally hide your Consciousness from your awareness), you do so to purge and neutralize all of what the Taoists call lower-level emotions: hatred, jealousy, depression, anger, viciousness, greed, vindictiveness, envy, and so on.

Post-Birth Considerations: Exorcising Ghosts

To become emotionally mature in Taoism you must also rid yourself of conditionings acquired after you were born. How many people can truthfully say they have gone beyond the way they were conditioned by their parents or other people and events from childhood? How many can see their parents, their brothers and sisters, and others they grew up with, including authority figures or subordinates, purely as human beings? How many people's relationships are played out with the partners reacting to each other and reliving the psychic wounds of their childhood? The Taoists maintain that in order to be spiritually prepared for having children, you need to evolve beyond (that is, release) negative conditioning that may have come from your parents.

Teachers in a variety of spiritual traditions recognize that all these influences from your past are like demons. In China, they call these traumas "internal demons" or "internal ghosts." First, you must become aware of the existence of such demons. Then, using the inner dissolving process as you dive into the core of your being, you literally disperse, release, and convert the "demon's" energy into spirit and emptiness.

A certain amount of courage is required for this journey. The Chinese call it "jumping into the dragon's mouth." You are going to get bitten. How strange it can feel when, in meditation, you encounter terrors stronger than anything you have experienced in your normal conscious life. At the level of the energy operating deep inside the mind, there is almost no difference experientially between events you consider to be real and memories that have no factual basis but are stored or created in what Western psychologists call the subconscious.

The Taoist methods for dissolving the demons inside the body are initiated by the mind systematically moving through the energy of the whole body, gaining the capacity over time to simultaneously dissolve the glands, brain, muscles, joints, and internal organs. Virtually all the cells of the body are scanned. The dissolving process finds energy clots and dismantles them, causing the previously blocked Chi to flow. It is not, however, only a question of getting rid of negative emotional and mental states, but of taking the free-flowing Chi and converting it to spirit.

A commonly overlooked point in some meditation traditions is that, if you wish to meditate solely to become physically and mentally relaxed, you run the risk of never gaining spirituality. People use chi gung for relaxing and avoiding depression, as if it were an antidepressant drug. Meditation can certainly calm or relax you, but its highest purpose in Taoism is to make you aware of the center of your being; that is, to find spirit and emptiness, the essential components of Consciousness itself. This level is beyond states of physical and mental relaxation; rather, it is relaxation into your being or "soul."

As long as you possess internal demons that either obsess or depress you, you cannot truly become fully internally relaxed; you cannot become natural; your innermost "soul" cannot relax. You must to some degree react to these inner emotions because they are etched into the various components of your being. All of us have personal emotional horror stories of greater or lesser severity. They are intrinsic to the human condition. All the Taoist meditation techniques systematically start releasing these internal demons where they have settled inside the body.

FOCUS ON A SPECIAL TOPIC
Releasing Internal Demons:
"My Back Will Never Recover"

 When I began to study martial arts at the age of twelve, I was stiff, uncoordinated, and disconnected from my body. When I asked my body to do something, it did not listen. Over the course of the next two decades, through many daily hours of vigorous training and self-discipline, my body changed. It became extremely flexible and strong and felt good all the time. Twenty years of hard work paid off—if I asked my body to do something, it did it with minimal resistance. All my boyhood dreams of having a body that worked well were fulfilled. My body became the instrument I used to express my artistic drives through high-level martial arts.

Then, in 1982, my body was severely damaged by a freak car accident. In thirty seconds, everything had been taken from me. My personal demon became fear reinforced by ever-present physical pain, fear that I would never recover, that my martial arts capacities were destroyed forever, that I was rendered incapable of doing the physical feats I had worked so hard to be able to take for granted. Whereas the first transformation brought joy, this one brought great pain and suffering—physical, emotional, and mental.

It gnawed at me that my body would never again be able to serve as an instrument of joy because of the aftereffects of a severely traumatized spine. After a while, the pain and body dysfunction improved a bit, and then got a whole lot worse. No matter how much I worked at rehabilitation, my condition progressively degenerated. My emotional frustrations and mood swings were like those of a musician going deaf.

For the next year and a half I worked hard to rebuild my body, but always some small movement would cause my back to destabilize. I would cycle again and again through anger to depression to hopelessness to resignation that I was slowly becoming a cripple. I limped when my back deteriorated. The intensity of the nerve pain in my spine increased month by month. Surgeons tried to convince me to go under the knife, but I resisted.

All my fears and terrors previously hidden within my body's energies and thus denied came out and plagued me like some animal tearing at my flesh. I went back to China,

FOCUS ON A SPECIAL TOPIC
Releasing Internal Demons:
"My Back Will Never Recover" (continued)

where my teacher Liu offered to help resolve this situation. He taught me chi gung and the Wu style of tai chi to heal my body and the sitting with internal dissolving method to release me from my inner demons. Whenever I got lazy in my practices, the incredible pain (which felt like an abscessed tooth inside my spinal cord) brought me back on track. The Wu style tai chi combined with the sitting dissolving method relieved the intense, grinding nerve pain. It also eased the emotional, mental, and psychic pain that had been released when my lifelong control and denial mechanisms were obliterated by the severe shock to my spine and its aftermath.

In the beginning of sitting, many days were devoted completely to releasing the physical pain. It is amazing how many different layers of defined nerve pain I found in my body. I dissolved the nerve pain of this part of my spine, then that part of my spine, of this energy and that energy, the pain that was lurking below the pain, and what was below that pain, ad infinitum. I knew that whatever I did not completely release at the next layer would plague me in a few hours. At that time, even a few hours of pain relief was a tremendous gift.

But the physical pain was not the worst of it. Even worse were those things that were deeper inside me: feelings of failure at not being able to conquer the pain, and the frustration of watching my body disintegrate. I found that as I dissolved and released physical pain, the process brought into clear focus every associated and hidden emotional trauma and fear repressed inside me. I used the relentless hurting on the physical level to unravel and expiate the pains and demons of my inner emotional, intellectual, and psychic world. It was rough.

When I practiced sitting and dissolving for upward of an hour or more, the physical and the emotional pain united. Previous emotional traumas, many from earliest childhood, had to be released in order for the physical pain to be released, and vice versa. It was one snake. I had mistakenly thought that the head and tail were intrinsically different, but the emotional and the physical were one interconnected whole.

I found specific connections between the pain and events from my personal history. Dissolving a pain in my midback,

FOCUS ON A SPECIAL TOPIC
Releasing Internal Demons:
"My Back Will Never Recover" (continued)

directly or indirectly through another thought, could bring me to an unresolved childhood trauma, to the failing of a test, or not getting something I really wanted, or the excessive pride or deep dejection associated with winning and losing. One pain turned into another. Releasing myself from attachments to useless things, such as pride, was especially difficult for me. Hopes, fears, desires granted and denied, repulsion, loneliness, pride, courage, generosity, greed, compassion, hatreds, jealousy. As these arose, I dissolved them all, all those emotional blocks that encrust and hide Consciousness from our living awareness.

Eventually, I reached the point where I could go through the layers, one by one, until the pain released into emptiness. Sometimes this left me with a brief physical respite and an inner peace that lasted for days. At other times, however, especially when the movement into emptiness was profound, demons released from the depths would revisit me with a vengeance. These forced me deeper and deeper into meditation, the only reliable means I had to relieve each new wave of psychic scorpions crawling over my heart and mind. After a while, my most intense demon, being rendered ineffective as a martial artist, vanished, and my focus shifted to that which was permanent: Consciousness itself.

Gradually, with Liu's help, I recovered physically, with my insides house-cleaned. This healing ultimately allowed me to rake away enough of the debris around my core to be able to see my Consciousness for what it was, clearly, on my own, in Canton, China, on a terribly rainy day.

FOCUS ON PRACTICE
Taoist Internal Breathing, Lesson 11:
Upper Back Breathing

You now want to combine both lower back breathing and full belly breathing with upper back breathing.

The lungs are constructed like a bag. If, when you inflate a bag, you hold the back of it still, the bag will inflate forward. This is how most people breathe, causing the chest to puff out, military style. If, however, you hold the front of the bag still, the bag will inflate backward. This is what we do with the chest in Taoist breathing.

The front of the chest (the sternum and chest muscles) completely relaxes and does not move at all, as the lungs expand backward toward the spine. As you do this, allow your shoulder blades to spread away from your spine and let your ribs and shoulders soften and move sideways. This action will release some of the anatomical bindings that prevent the lungs from fully expanding backward to their utmost capacity.

Two forces now simultaneously combine to give your heart a continuous massage with each breath, which is absent or diminished in regular puffed-out chest breathing: (1) the spreading of the ribs, shoulder blades, and shoulders causes greater movement in back of the heart, and (2) upward pressure is applied to the heart by the diaphragm. These two directional forces compress and release the heart muscle and pericardium in a tonifying, rhythmic massage.

This heart massage, combined with the lower belly breathing's massage of your other internal organs, now tonifies and increases blood circulation to all your internal organs.

Begin with two breaths and gradually work up to thirty breaths combining lower back (kidney) breathing, full belly front and sides breathing, and upper back breathing.

Emotional Maturity from the Taoist View

As you go through and release the energy inside yourself, you start to become mature. The difference between mature people and children is that children are always quite sure of how things ought to be. They are quite clear about the way life must be, should be, has got to be, and if it isn't that way, they sulk or throw tantrums.

A mature human being is one who finally realizes that quite a few things are just how they are. Mature individuals can relax and function well amid life's imperfections, without the need to be recognized or to condemn. They can forgive people. They can accept that people have limitations and generally do what they are able to do. Through the maturity practices, the Taoist meditator moves toward a personal freedom from conditioned emotions and thought patterns. The freedom may take years of practice to obtain, because it is not easy to grow up. But once you have accomplished this task, you are ready to start working with your spirituality—for you will have reached the state where you can begin Taoist alchemical work, where all your energies are fully ready to be converted to spirit, emptiness, and ultimately, the Tao.

In the intermediate stage of Taoist meditation, you dissolve the internal organs and then the glands. A major goal is to be able to free the energy of your glands, which can lead you to experience either violent or subtle emotions. Your glands contribute routinely to all aspects of your physiology and therefore to your mental states. What we think of as emotions are often in reality our neural transmitters, organs, or glands relocating energy.

All the emotions in the body can, through Taoist meditation, be converted to their opposites. Anger can be turned into love, fear to courage. This conversion is accomplished through many generic and individualized meditative practices.

You can undergo various internal energetic changes by doing such practices as intentionally switching the energy from one organ to the next, linking it to the depths of your mind, purposefully playing with the energy that is inside your spine, and working with the many energy centers inside the brain.* As you do so, you become able to liberate the basic negative conditionings that prevent maturity—in

---

*Working with the energy centers of the brain is a dangerous practice for beginners and should be done only under the guidance of an authentic master.

other words, all of the negative things that make life painful, difficult, and problematic. Next comes what is even more challenging: you must clear out attachments for everything you like. Why? So you can let things be what they are without either positive or negative events in the world influencing your consciousness.

It is quite easy, when you experience trauma, to take an attitude of "woe is me," or "I'm angry," or "I'm sad," or "I'm depressed." In the Taoist way, it is necessary to transform such emotions to neutral energy. Most people can relate to this kind of freedom. But what about when you start doing away with things that you like most in the world? What about the issue of dissipating the attachments to everything you passionately desire and yet retaining the ability to feel fully alive and actively engaged? Here, indeed, is a formidable challenge that has troubled everyone who has attained the Tao.

As you begin this challenge, you are still taking responsibility for your practice. What you have to do is first work on things that bother you the most and then assume responsibility for the totality of what is inside you, warts and all.

You may take responsibility for your practice, but this act alone does not indicate entirely taking responsibility truly for who you are. In one sense, your practice can simply be selfish and self-motivated. My hand is hurting me; I just want it to stop hurting. This does not necessarily mean that I take responsibility for my hand. It may only mean that I don't want to be in pain—a perfectly valid motivation, but one that alone will not lead me to the Tao. To move further toward the Tao, you need to understand and transcend everything to do with your hand, both the good and the bad, to truly take responsibility for your Consciousness.

Being Unattached Does Not Mean Being Incapable of Action

Some people have the mistaken idea that anyone who is nonattached and spiritually clear loses all passion for life, ceases caring about anything. The attitude is that nonattached people can't do anything, will dissolve away the will to fight evil or will rid themselves of compassion for the needy. Nothing could be more erroneous. Examples abound of "nonattached" people engaging in action: the gentle Jesus Christ threw the money changers out of the temple in Jerusalem; Buddhist monks burned themselves to death in Vietnam to passively resist the war. Sun Tsu's Taoist classic *The Art of War* is a tactical manual for action. The Indian classic *Bhagavad Gita*, wherein Arjuna is told by the god Krishna to make war with his relatives in a nonattached fashion, is another good example. Both of these works frown on the blind uselessness of war, but if it must be waged for good reasons (such as against Hitler's Germany), these writings explain how to take action and expertly fight the forces of evil.

Chi is the force of life. The more Chi you have, the more life you have, the more passion you have. The outer passion and creativity of the artist and the inner passion and creativity of the meditator are flip sides of the same coin. Many cultures glorify a passion for life. In the West, the great novel *Zorba the Greek* by Nikos Kazantzakis epitomizes this quality, as does the French phrase *joie de vivre*. Genuine passion means to be truly in the moment, fully engaged, and wanting to be nowhere else. It is a personality trait, an attitude toward life. Different people have different things they are naturally drawn to and through which they express their passion. The genuinely passionate will be as equally engaged in fighting evil as in promoting good, in having fun or in deferring it. Passion brings joy, regardless of the content of our interest. It is different from those endless compulsive churnings of the mind that drive people but leave them dry inside, in the fruitless need to succeed or be right.

If "non-attachment" is based strictly on philosophy (that is, you *ought* to be non-attached, just as you *ought* not to sin), most people will never become authentically non-attached. Natural selfish needs will invariably put them at loggerheads with their philosophy. The wise Taoists were humble enough to realize that the universe moves in unknowable ways. They believed that unless you have the wisdom to foresee how all the interconnections of events unfold across time and space, it's okay to want, but foolish to get upset by being attached to results.

Many stories in Asia concerning the virtues of non-attachment tell with innumerable variations of individuals who have wonderful good fortune and rant and rave about it. Times change, as they always do, and the result of the good fortune creates a disaster. The disaster then creates good fortune. Bad fortune, good fortune—the story is usually told in five to ten cycles. All the while the protagonist cries and beats his chest, "Oh, how wonderful is my good fortune"; "Oh, woe is me for my bad fortune." The lessons of the stories are always that attachment may or may not be what it's cracked up to be when you take into account the world's never-ending change.

The Taoist phrase connoting non-attachment is *wu wei*, or "doing without doing." Non-attachment to the ultimate disposition of things enables you to act quietly or passionately on your feelings and convictions without reservation. And yet the source of that passion is not your convoluted neurosis or ego inflation, but the Consciousness shining through you for purposes that ultimately may be beyond most people's wisdom to understand in the moment. You do nothing; Consciousness itself does. Right-wing Taoists usually retire to the mountains, as they feel their time for activity in the striving world is completed. They reserve their passion for meditating alone. Left-wing Taoists are often passionately and actively engaged with balancing and ameliorating evils (as they perceive them) and promoting good in the world.

FOCUS ON PRACTICE

Taoist Internal Breathing, Lesson 12:
Breathing Energy into the Tantien

 Continue to practice everything you have
learned from Lessons 1 through 11. Now add
breathing into your tantien.

Your lower tantien is located down from your
navel about one-third of the distance to your
genitals, just slightly above your pubic hair, in
the center of your abdomen, midway between the surface of
the skin of your belly and your spine, on the central channel.
It is the only energetic center in your body that controls and
regulates every energy that affects your physical health. You
want to find this place in your body by feeling for it rather
than visualizing it. This energy center has an initially fuzzy
and eventually clear sensation, distinct from everything
around it. It cannot be physically seen by your eyes, although
it can be energetically felt or even psychically seen by a sufficiently trained or sensitive individual.

The lower tantien may be felt as either a tiny point or a
small ball. The tantien is the center of a sea of energy. In the
West it is probably best known by its Japanese name, the *hara*.

Imagine energy moving in and out with your breath and
feel yourself breathing into your tantien in four progressive
steps, achieving effortlessness in one step before moving on to
the next.

Step 1. In the front of your body, inhale from your skin to
your tantien and exhale from your tantien to your skin. Next,
breathe in energy from your etheric body—the space three to
six inches outside your physical body—backward into your
tantien. Exhale from your lower tantien, through your physical body, past your physical body, and back to where you
originally inhaled from your etheric body. The continuous
conscious awareness of your mindstream should now be
moving past a sense of physical matter into your chi body.

The acupuncture point called the *ming men*, or "door of
life," is located on the spine directly behind the tantien. It is
often called the back tantien. Besides being a primary control
point for the elimination of lower back pain and for enabling
movement of energy along the spine, it is also the energetic
control point for the kidneys, which are the source of vitality
and thereby life of the human body. The ming men opens up
the life force in a person, and hence its name.

FOCUS ON PRACTICE
Taoist Internal Breathing, Lesson 12:
Breathing Energy into the Tantien (continued)

Step 2. Inhale from the ming men point to your lower tantien. Now exhale from the tantien to ming men. Build progressively to thirty complete breaths.

Step 3. Fuse steps 1 and 2 together. Inhale simultaneously from both the front and back. In front, inhale from the boundary of your etheric body at the point just beyond your tantien; in back, inhale from the etheric boundary just beyond the ming men. With this inhale, bring breath energy from both directions simultaneously through your etheric body, skin, and flesh into your lower tantien. Upon exhaling, allow the breath energy to exit simultaneously in a straight line from your tantien, through to your etheric body both in the front and in the back. This will activate the *dai mai*.

The dai mai is an extraordinary acupuncture meridian that encircles the body from the tantien to the door of life—ming men—and back to the tantien. It holds a special place in the body's energy system. The dai mai belt meridian intersects with, connects, and integrates all the body's twelve main vertical acupuncture meridians. At first, by breathing through from the tantien to the ming men, you activate the dai mai, energizing all your other acupuncture meridians simultaneously.* The energy lines inside your body, as well as your external aura to the edge of your etheric body, are directly connected to each other in a circular relationship, one activating the other. When your tantien breathing continues past your skin to the edge of your etheric body or aura, it connects the two primary (front and back) points on your external aura and thus activates, integrates, and strengthens your whole aura. When your auric energy is activated, it reinforces the strengths of your acupuncture meridian lines. This strengthening forms the door through which you can progressively become aware of the energy in your whole aura.

This Taoist breathing method was also historically used in Chinese Chan Buddhism but was not passed down to Zen Buddhism in Japan or, for that matter, to the Japanese martial arts community, including aikido. It performs two functions simultaneously: (a) it makes the body sensitive, healthy, and strong, and (b) it extends your conscious awareness from your

*This includes the governor and conception vessels, which are also called the microcosmic orbit.

FOCUS ON PRACTICE
Taoist Internal Breathing, Lesson 12:
Breathing Energy into the Tantien (continued)

physical body to your chi. Consequently, your ability to be consciously aware of what is happening in your mindstream for long periods of time is expanded.

Gradually build tantien to ming men breathing from two to thirty breaths.

Step 4. This is truly an optional step that should be done only after step 3 completely stabilizes. If you do not have extensive experience with energy work, it is best to stick to practicing step 3 for a minimum of three months before progressing to step 4.

As this stabilization occurs, the subtle sensation of the breath moving back and forth along the line between your etheric body and tantien should have the clearly felt sensation of being connected and unbroken. After this occurs the dai mai will automatically activate. As your awareness grows through practice, the felt sensation of the encircling dai mai should progressively become more clear, both on your skin and in your etheric body. Being able to feel the dai mai will make it significantly easier for you to both increase its strength and consciously join its energy to your tantien.

> (a) Inhale and breathe energy from the entire circumference of the dai mai on your skin, through your body, and into your tantien. Exhale and return the breath energy from your tantien, through your body, and to the entire circumference of the dai mai on your skin.

> (b) Inhale, and from the dai mai's entire circum-ference in your etheric body, breathe energy through the air, to your skin, and through your body into your tantien. Exhale, and reversing the same pathway, breathe energy from your tantien, through your body, to the entire dai mai's circumference on your skin, and through the air to the dai mai's entire circumference in your etheric body.

The Deeper Challenges of Taoist Meditation

CHAPTER
8

I Ching : Hexagram 51–Thunder

Thunder comes, extending its terror far and wide
Its shock brings forth success, then joy
Now is the time to be aware of the sacred
As the Tao comes forth in Thunder

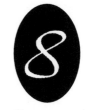

The Deeper Challenges of Taoist Meditation

The Center of Your Awareness: *Hsin,* or Heart-Mind

In the intermediate stage of meditative practice, at some point you start dealing with the interesting question, Where is the origin of thought? You begin to move into an area the Chinese call the *hsin,* or heart-mind, which is on the edge of alchemy, or energy transformation. You are not quite fully immersed in alchemy yet, but are getting there. At this level of meditation, you start working with the techniques of the heart and mind, which allow your awareness to begin to perceive the place where thoughts originate. You discover what your thought actually is, and you become acutely aware of the consciousness that generates your thought. You take the first steps that move you toward the center of your being.

Most of us right now can recognize the existence of thought, of something in your head, be it scientific, intellectual, or philosophical pondering, or else the mundane: I know that two plus two equals four; I am doing the laundry tomorrow morning; I am going to buy some milk on the way home; and so on. Ordinary thinking represents a certain type of mental activity that virtually everyone will acknowledge is present.

But when you start going to that place where the consciousness that literally travels from birth to death is generated, you have reached the middle ground of meditation work. This is where you start dealing with

Consciousness. The cellular-level dissolving techniques tend to be important until you reach the stage where you can start dissolving through the mind flow, and then through the emotions, until eventually you find where thought is actually being produced. You literally follow the mindstream to the edge of the direct experience of Consciousness itself.

When your conscious awareness arrives at this destination, you can start using all sorts of techniques to unravel the shapes, or knots, in your consciousness. The major effect of this part of the meditation training is to give you awareness of the core of your being in order to accustom you to working with it. Any individual approaching the core of his or her being can panic. When getting close to the core, most run like hell or scream. (If you are lucky, you only scream.) Usually, people simply cut off and become absolutely numb. There is a good reason for this: fear of the death of the ego.

Ru Ding: Fear of the Death of the Ego

One of the great psychological difficulties that practitioners encounter in Taoist meditation is the fear that comes from losing one's ego. This fear leaves a person feeling a total loss of control. The Chinese call the experience of this primal fear *ru ding*. When ru ding occurs (either during standing, sitting, moving, lying down, or sexual practices), a total fear grips every part of your being. It is not that you are consciously afraid of something in particular, as if someone were trying to physically or emotionally injure you; rather, an amorphous, nonspecific fear paralyzes you right down to the center of your being, pervading every cell of your body and every crevice of your mind. You are in a complete state of terror, face to face with panic and anxiety without cause or reason. Your central nervous system may well find this psychic pain unbearable—you just want to shut down so you cannot feel it, even though you do not know where it is coming from.

If you can stay in it, every second geometrically amplifies the internal intensity of the formless pain. Your cells scream to "get out of here," yet it is only by remaining in the intensity of this most distressing emotional and psychic event that you can go permanently through it and come out the other side, for if you do not get through it, it will only recur.

Most Taoist meditators, when initially experiencing ru ding, do not know what has hit them. They do not understand what is going on, only that whatever it is, it scares the stuffing out of them and they hope it will never come back. Sadly, this experience can, by force of will, be suppressed. When this suppression occurs, it causes a serious, insurmountable spiritual obstacle to the process of meditation and internal freedom.

THE WAY OF LIU
The Horror of the Loss of the Ego

 I was in Hong Kong beginning to learn the old Yang style of tai chi chuan when ru ding first struck me out of the blue. It was late at night, at a still and quiet terrace on the Peak, where few people came after midnight. Finding a quiet, solitary place with clean air and some greenery to practice in severely crowded Hong Kong is no easy task. Every once in a while a gentle breeze rustled the trees, breaking the dead silence of the night in this tiny park. When the breeze died down, the park became quiet, and the moon and the sky felt as though they were descending downward, putting enormous pressure on every square inch of my skin, as I tried to lift my arms with the expansive energy of tai chi. However, no matter how much my energy pushed out, I felt as if the Chi from the moonlight, stars, and sky penetrated my body against my will. My body and mind became immensely still, as though they had dropped into a bottomless abyss, even though I was doing the rhythmic slow motion movements of tai chi.

At the depth of the stillness, an overwhelming, formless fear began to develop in my belly. I persevered, but each movement became progressively harder, as if the sky had

THE WAY OF LIU

The Horror of the Loss of the Ego (continued)

turned into steel and was encasing my body, blocking its ability to move.

Then it happened: an all-consuming, paralyzing fear seemed all at once to invade every cell in my body. My tai chi movements slowed dramatically, to what felt like an inch an hour. Sweat began immediately to pour out of my groin, legs, hands, face, back, my entire body. The fear grew exponentially. My nerves and energy channels felt as if they would shatter—my very right to existence was being stripped away for no apparent reason. I knew if I kept practicing there would be nothing left of me in a few seconds. The fear was absolutely irrational yet real beyond belief, alive, vibrant, terrifying. I stopped practicing the tai chi and ran down the hill, praying hard that this terror would leave me. And suddenly it did.

Later, in Beijing, Liu explained to me that the nature of ru ding was about fear of losing your ego, rather than merely the loss of the physical body, which could be replaced by means of reincarnation. The fear of physical death alone will not activate ru ding. However, moving into an awareness of the nonseparation of yourself and the whole of existence can cause this horrendous inner fear to arise. The Taoists believe that the energies in the human soul/consciousness that can move from living entity to living entity do not consider the physical shell (body) to be of any consequence to their survival. If the body dies, they continue, through reincarnation.

The universal energy that connects all of creation is called *yuan chi* in Chinese. The ego, or the sense of separation, goes into mortal fear when the false reality of being separate from the universal life force (yuan chi) is threatened by your consciousness having reached an awareness of its connection to everything in existence. The ego then spews forth all sorts of terrifying psychological and physical reactions in the body and mind to make meditators petrified of leaving the state of separation, or to addict them to the psychic energies of the separation. Through this ego process, meditators are encouraged to move as far away from merging with the energy of existence as possible, thereby allowing the ego to defend itself and survive.

While rationally it makes perfect sense to want to become free of the pain that causes ego, at the psychic level the reality

THE WAY OF LIU

The Horror of the Loss of the Ego (continued)

is far different. The fear evoked begins at the causal energy level and is amplified at the psychic level until almost all of your physical, emotional, and intellectual awareness is thoroughly terrorized. Ru ding is an experience in traditional spirituality where the ego and the higher capacities of a human being fight for dominance. It might be compared to what in Christianity is called "the dark night of the soul." Liu pointed out that in Taoism, ru ding can be a stepping stone to a meditator's eventually unifying with the Tao, as well as part of the price paid for the journey.

Unfortunately, there is no quick cure for ru ding, no one magic practice that will get you through it quickly. How long this experience lasts or how many times it recurs is a matter of both the strength and tenacity of your karma and how much you will need to understand this phenomenon. After the battle with the ego and separation has been positively resolved, and you find out who you are, this understanding can allow you to pass through ru ding and come out to be a positive, compassionate force for balance in the fabric of interconnected life.

In the Eastern meditative traditions, meditators are believed to have spent numerous lives working toward enlightenment, not to mention an especially intense decade or two, or even five, in the final life when they actually become clear. The experience of ru ding rarely happens to people until they are in the final rounds of the protracted battle for their inner essence. Ru ding functions to make meditators aware that they have more serious spiritual work to do—it is a kind of a spiritual wake-up call. At a very powerful psychic level, it reminds you of the visceral grief your ego is causing you. It motivates you to practice with renewed vigor, as you will do almost anything to keep it from returning. When ru ding does return, it tends to clear away any delusions about how wonderfully your spiritual work has been progressing. A well-known Taoist saying about ru ding is: "It helps the fool become wise. Especially when the fool gets drowsy and begins to fall asleep." If you can become pragmatically aware of your ego, you can systematically work toward ridding yourself of its burden. Ru ding is consequently considered a blessing for self-awareness rather than a worldly curse.

THE WAY OF LIU
Ferocity of the Ego

 Liu used this analogy concerning ru ding: There is a house cat (that is, your emotions) that you want to stroke and make your friend. You approach it too suddenly, however, and scare it. It hisses and tries to scratch you. Because it is only a small house cat, you can, if you choose, grab it by the scruff of the neck and force your will on it.

The ego, though, is no small tabby. It is more like a four-hundred-pound tiger that can kill or maim you with one swipe of its paw. One must approach a cat like this gingerly, with respect. When you initially move toward the tiger from fifty feet, its first roar will scare you almost to death. You will run. The next approach, gentle if you please, may with luck get you within forty feet of the tiger before it roars at you. Still, terror will ripple through you and you will retreat. You will play this cat-and-mouse game with the tiger, getting closer and retreating in cycles, each time becoming more sensitive to the tiger's moves and moods. After repeated attempts, you let it know that you are its friend. Eventually, the tiger will let you get close enough to touch it. Then, ultimately, it will begin to purr. At this point, exercise caution, because the tiger can suddenly turn mean. But if it stays tame, play with it gently. Then, in all likelihood, the tiger will not bother you again.

Until the final round, your ego will get increasingly more deceptive, subtle, and devious to protect its survival. It is at these points that you must be most careful and maintain your genuine humility and spiritual integrity. Although the fear of losing your ego is temporarily terrifying, it is, Liu emphasized, an experience that many on the spiritual path need to undergo as a positive source of growth, whether they choose to or not.

The Next Level: Manifestation

Once you have gained access to the core of your consciousness, you begin practices to explore your own psychic energy as well as that of others, and to realize that your psychic body extends into time and space. There then arises the question of a thing called *manifestation*. Where do things come from and why have they manifested in a particular way? Why do you dress as you do now rather than in robes or furs, or why are you sitting down at this moment instead of dancing on the roof? Why does this world exist when it could also not exist? This world had to come into being in some way. You had to come into existence some way. The thought you hold for the next second comes from somewhere. At this level of Taoist meditation, you learn to understand and work with the unseen world.

Caution: In all traditions this is a dangerous time, requiring the meditator to engage in extremely deep soul-searching. At this juncture, the subtle yet powerful frailties of the human ego tend to emerge from the darker recesses of our innermost selves.

Here you start dealing with the cause of manifestation—in other words, the source of where everything you know comes from. In this psychic stage, your mind will reach out farther and farther from your physical body, in a process that enables you to recognize energetic cause-and-effect relationships that are not ordinarily accessible through the rational mind.

It is as though, in New York City, something stirs on 59th Street, then moves down and down, and when it finally arrives at First Street, it manifests. But as an advanced Taoist meditator, you have started tapping into the capacity to discern what this energy is when it commences transforming in earnest up at 42nd Street and how it differs when it congeals and arrives at 23rd Street. This period of practice usually destabilizes people involved in Taoist meditation—they lose recognizable landmarks. The world now ceases to be so solid for them. It takes time to recognize the new guideposts of the psychic world, for a sense of "reality" to develop on that plane. Energy becomes the same as matter to you. Acclimation is necessary.

Your energy is churning about, and there is a questioning of what is real and what is not, which is characterized in Taoism as "learning to discriminate between the real and the false." This phase is difficult for meditators; at this point, most people not only start learning how to get the message but also begin to grasp the mechanics. How can you stop things before they hit you? How can you play with and manipulate these energies in order to transform your mind until it is still and unmoving? You go beyond being influenced by the energies. This is not magic. It does, however, require a consistent and long-term effort.

Taoism, as it has descended from Lao Tse, never intends to use psychic knowledge for purposes of power in the world of manifestation, but only to increase internal awareness in order to free yourself from internal prisons built of "red dust." Some Taoists, the magicians in fire approaches, do play with the energies of the psychic and causal planes to control the environment of the mental, emotional, chi, and physical planes. In terms of meditation, you can manipulate environments for all you are worth to get worldly rewards, but you (that is, your soul, that which the Taoists maintain is deathless and can reincarnate) will still be energetically trapped within that environment if you don't get past desiring the power. Sooner or later you will fall from your elevated state of spiritual grace as a result of misusing your new powers. Herein is the real problem. With the ability to know what you will know—foreknowledge of what will happen in the future, the ability to cause or manipulate events, and so on—you must consider all of these phenomena and clearly understand at this point that you are just a player in the game, not the creator of the game. Any delusion of your being an all-powerful creator eventually leads to spiritual egomania, rendering you incapable of eventually becoming completely clear. This is a trap that many actual or aspiring "gurus" can all too easily fall into. You are simply hearing about the news before it arrives. The fact is that for everything you can perceive that might turn into a wonderful thing, there is also potential for it to become a disaster.

At this stage, you start to enter into practices that the Chinese call *nei dan*. Now that you have some awareness of these energies coming down from the causal plane (that is, the source of manifestation), you will have to deliberately rewire (or transmute) your system to be able to allow the energies to pass through you without your being affected and without your affecting them. When these psychic forces come down, most of us are powerfully influenced by them. It is a great temptation to want to play with them, to use your will to make them behave how you want them to. It takes great internal strength to leave them be, a position that is part of the noninterference doctrine of the Tao. It is extremely hard to be humble enough to allow existence to operate without your influence when you have the power to manipulate it.

This phase of meditative practice, whether you are on the way of fire or water, is tricky. At the resolution of this stage, stillness naturally arises. This stillness continues, through meditation, to be refined until you reach the Great Stillness, which causes all the separate parts of your being to conjoin in a unified whole and you find out truly who you are. In many traditions, this state is termed *enlightenment.*

At this point and afterward, the process of alchemy transfigures your vibrational level to higher and higher frequencies, bringing you into direct, permanent contact with the underlying energy of the universe—the Tao. Once you reach the Tao, all discomfort ceases.

THE WAY OF LIU
The Root of the Mind

 In 1985 I took a two-week trip to see my family in America. While I was there, my beloved grandfather died, ending a major chapter of my life. En route back to Beijing, I landed in Hong Kong. A forecasted typhoon forced me to leave earlier than planned for Canton, the next destination before flying to Beijing. Arriving in Canton in the morning, with a day to spare before my flight, I obtained a bed in an eight-bed dormitory room, next to a window. The other beds were occupied by Chinese travelers. My sparse finances at the time did not allow me a room to myself.

The hotel had no restaurant. I sat and meditated for about eight hours, dissolving into some of the deepest spaces I had ever gone into. The rain intensified all day; the dirt road from the hotel to the restaurants became progressively muddier. I had dinner, watching the hard rain, bought some light snacks, and went back to the room to begin meditating again. The meditations became deeper and stronger. I meditated till three o'clock in the morning.

My plane was scheduled to leave at one o'clock in the afternoon, but the flight was canceled because of the storm. The rain did not let up, and the mud got deeper and deeper.

That afternoon I began one of the most intense meditation sessions I had ever had. It continued until the next morning, nonstop. Each dissolving experience was progressively more intense with ever more vivid internal sounds, three-dimensional visions, smells, and energetic sensations. Each time I went through one layer of my mind, the resulting sense of emptiness and space inside and outside me got larger, penetrating right inside my very cells. As the inner experiences intensified, the resulting release created an ever-deepening and all-encompassing silence.

As these releases happened, I gradually gained a glimpse of this thing that was there and never left, even as the experiences themselves became more and more overpowering. As the night turned to day, I was finding myself dissolving elements from both the past, present, and future, discovering all of them to have equal impact, as though there was no difference. At one point, after an extremely powerful release, I clearly saw with complete relaxation this "thing" that before I had only glimpsed, the thing that was always there no matter what sensations or experiences my mind was consciously

THE WAY OF LIU
The Root of the Mind (continued)

aware of. It seemed that all the content of my mind, my personal history, events, experiences, beliefs, traumas, joys, attachments, aversions, perceptions, were just like suspended particles. They had no cohesion. They were not who I was. It was clear that this "thing," this fluid that everything was attaching to, was permanent and had always been there, regardless of what else was going on. It was there now and most likely would always be there. All the mind business, emotions and perceptions included, was just "stuff" floating in suspension. And yet all my life I had taken the stuff so seriously, certain that the stuff was me. In one swift moment it became clear that it was not me. Rather, I was the fluid, the ground, that which is changeless and existing under all conditions and times, the solution the stuff was floating in, the permanence that was truly me, and clearly not the stuff, which had ruled and dominated every second of my life until that moment.

I found the absurdity of confusing the "stuff" inside me for who I am, and all the nonsense this confusion had caused me in my life, to be enormously funny—the cosmic joke, which I and almost every other human being had been focusing on, taking so seriously all our lives. How this confusion of something so simple and basic caused so much internal pain and frustration in myself and, I was sure, in many of those I had met throughout my life became undeniably obvious.

The humor of this cosmic joke got to me at such a deep level that I could not stop laughing, even through the unpleasant mud and rain. For the next few days, until I took the plane back to Beijing, I laughed. For most of my life before this I was a relatively humorless person, who concentrated on the intensity of my own and other people's "stuff." After Canton, a sense of humor developed in me. Slowly but surely I no longer took myself, or life in general seriously. During these few days waiting for the plane, each time I meditated, the internal stillness deepened until it implanted itself in my being as a permanent structure.

In Beijing, Liu told me before I even spoke that I had made some small progress and asked what happened. I told him, and he pointed out that I had seen the root of my mind and had become stable there. He said this was a first major step. My experiencing the Great Stillness, he said, was like cutting the root of the mind, the root of the tree, upon which

THE WAY OF LIU
The Root of the Mind (continued)

hung the "stuff." Even though the root was cut, it would take about ten years for the tree to completely die and all the accumulated energy of the tree to finish its natural cycles. The work of the Great Stillness, however, was done. Now, Liu said, it was time to begin learning Taoist meditation's final phase of internal alchemy, now that I had cut the root of my heart-mind and was continuously aware that that which does not change is the material of which Consciousness is made. Liu said, "First rest for a while and become comfortable and relaxed in this new way of relating to life. Then, after you settle down, let's move into learning about internal alchemy." Which we did until he died.

Frequently Asked Questions
About Taoist Meditation

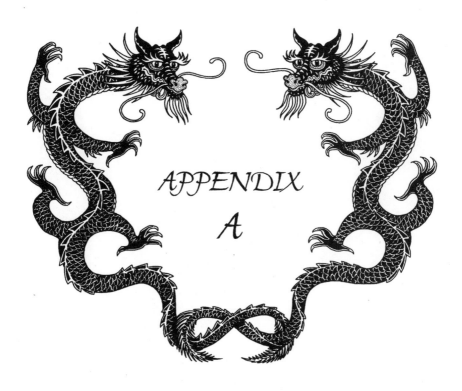

APPENDIX

A

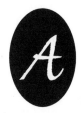

Frequently Asked Questions about Taoist Meditation

1. *In the standing and moving practices, how do you deal with the mental and physical strain than can come from maintaining the required body alignments?*

By practicing consistently and applying the 70 percent rule (see Chapter 1). At each stage of practice, you fluctuate between releasing nerve tension, releasing your habitually shortened small muscles, and stabilizing your mind, all without straining past your limits. Habitual tension fatigues your nerves and shortens your muscles. Tension that has taken decades to harden like cement in your body will take time to dissipate.

Habitual tension, which virtually everyone in our technological society suffers from, weakens the stamina of the nerves that inform your body parts how to maintain proper physical alignment in order to maximize the energy flows in your channels. When your nerves are tired and you force them to perform beyond their capacity, you feel the result as strain and pain. In the many important small muscles needed to comfortably maintain proper physical alignments, cumulative habitual tension within the nerves induces permanent muscular contractions, both overt and subtle. Acquired over years, these habitual contractions shorten the natural length of the small muscles, as well as their associated ligaments and tendons. Shortened muscles add to the aches and pains of maintaining the alignments, as your body is being asked to stretch beyond its current ability in a manner similar to the strain that comes from being forced to do a leg split. Shortened muscles are also responsible for back, neck, and shoulder pain, nearly an epidemic in modern cultures.

The vicious downward spiral goes like this: tension activates the nerves, which signal the muscles to contract, which further shortens the muscles, pulling on the insertion points where they attach to bones and ligaments, which causes fatigue and strain, which causes blood circulation to diminish in the area, which blocks the chi in your energy channels. The blocked chi causes pain, which causes more tension, and the whole downward spiral continuously repeats, ad infinitum.

Now let's look at two necessary activities that can reverse the situation: Achieving softness allows the muscles to stretch and the nerves to release, and therefore lessens tension. Achieving relaxation without collapsing yields softness and a mind that is stable and comfortable with a certain degree of physical stretch, as well as increasing nerve strength so that the nerves can maintain a smooth flow of energy.

Softness comes from lengthening your habitually contracted shortened muscles and tendons. Relaxation comes from mentally letting go of habitual tension in the nerves, by means of the dissolving process. When the nerves relax, their stamina and strength increase. You need strength of nerves to be able to tell your muscles to continuously and gently lengthen in the necessary ways. Nerve strength, not muscular strength, is required for you to be able remain upright. Weight lifters, gymnasts, and others of immense muscular strength have the same problems maintaining soft relaxed alignments as do nonmuscular types. Nerve relaxation causes your muscles to relax. Once deep relaxation occurs, the weight of these soft tissues and associated fluids (that is, blood, lymph, and so on) will gradually and gently pull on your other soft tissues, including ligaments, tendons, and especially fascia. This gentle pulling without tension gradually stretches soft tissues and thereby lengthens them.

Large stretching movements are effective on big muscles but not the tiny muscles that are bound up with fascia. While a bound piece of fascia is in the process of stretching to its natural length, you may feel discomfort or strain. The fascia and shortened muscles and tendons will stretch in increments, with plateaus that need time to be traversed before advancing to the next increment. They will not stretch out instantaneously. If they were forced to, they would be likely to tear.

How quickly nerves will relax and subsequently strengthen, as well as how rapidly your shortened muscles will stretch, cannot be predicted; it depends on each individual. All of us have differing genetic makeups and varying degrees of sensitivity and talent in connecting with internal subtle sensations. The presence or absence of trauma can also affect the rate of the process. What can be said for sure is that the more you regularly do the preliminary practices following the 70 percent rule, the faster the results, and vice versa.

Therefore, you must find your own personal balance between (a) mentally and emotionally letting go of the tension in your nerves, and (b) letting your soft tissues stretch to the new next stage (for example, while lifting your spine or your midriff or dropping your chest). When you have reached a new level, stay there for however many days it takes for your mind to stabilize. Until you have attained stabilization and comfort, do not attempt to stretch even a tiny bit more. It is this trying to go the little bit more—breaking the 70 percent rule—that results in the strain and stress. The tension resulting from the strain in turn prevents the body and mind from relaxing and softening.

Once one alignment has become stabilized and easy for you to achieve without concentration, you may then add another, so that you are doing two different alignments simultaneously. Follow the same procedure until the two are stabilized, then add a third, doing all three at the same time, and so on. Again, the importance of stabilizing at each stage before adding something new must be emphasized. As the chain of alignments you have mastered grows, you may find that an earlier link was not as stable as you thought. Return and rebuild the weak link by again releasing the nerves, restretching the shortened tissue, and stabilizing the mind. Then rebuild the entire chain, from the beginning, without weak links, all over again. If all the other links were solid, this rebuilding process should take only a few seconds, or at most minutes. If another weak link appears, work on it with the same procedure before moving forward.

The point of balance lies in not putting expectations on yourself that exceed your natural limits in the pursuit of perfection. Going beyond your limits ultimately leads to "three steps forward and two steps back," an undesirable approach. Slow and steady is what wins this race.

2. *Is it dangerous to practice water method meditation while using prescription drugs?*

The prescription drugs of allopathic medicine, along with herbal or homeopathic remedies, are normally used to ameliorate some kind of disease. To the best of my knowledge, practicing Taoist meditation while taking any of these medicines is safe insofar as physiologically based problems are concerned. Taoist meditation has for millennia been used to restore health or to enhance the medical procedures of massage, acupuncture, and bone setting and the herbal remedies found in traditional Chinese medicine. This tradition continues in China today, as hospitals apply tai chi, chi gung, and methods of meditation to a great variety of physical problems. In these hospitals, both traditional Chinese medicine and Western allopathic medicine, including drugs and surgery, complement each other and are integrated to obtain maximum benefit for the patient.

The experience in China has been that the water methods of meditation, being sufficiently gentle, are safe; however, there are cautions, such as in the case of drug-specific dangers from a substance that can lower or raise blood pressure. To be absolutely certain, consult your physician. If dangers exist in the fire methods of Taoist meditation they are generally to be found in excessively forceful practices that encourage cathartic vibrating or intense body shaking, holding of the breath, or muscular contractions.

The question of the impact on one's mental health is another story. I know of no in-depth research or experience to indicate how combining any method of meditation with drugs used for mental illnesses would affect someone with a mental disorder. Tai chi, however, has been used positively to treat the post-traumatic stress disorders of Vietnam veterans.

3. *Is it dangerous to practice water method meditation while on recreational drugs?*

Taoists believe that recreational drugs dull clarity of mind and thereby retard or completely block progress toward the deeper levels of meditation. True, you can point to a large variety of cultures worldwide that have employed any number of mind-altering drugs to enter into psychic realms. Some of these drugs are integral parts of solid spiritual traditions, but are not part of the water method of Taoism, which purely uses the five modes of practice (see Chapter 5) without external support.

Having said that, there are some things to consider. We live in a world where drugs are rampant, including alcohol and tobacco. Many who use one drug or another also meditate. A Taoist would typically look at this reality and ponder the practical ramifications involved.

Many young people try recreational drugs to experience the "something more" that they feel is inside themselves but to which they have no access. The use of hallucinogens, for example, often provides the drug taker an expanded internal experience of the possibilities of the body-mind. Such mind/spirit expansions are potentially good, but exploring them with drugs may extract a terrible price. Drug-induced visions, moreover, are not even a remote shadow of what the spirit and Consciousness have to offer a human being.

Once drug users learn through Taoist meditation to go inside and find the living spiritual root that dwells there (however slowly they do this, as the drugs will impede their progress), they just might reduce their intake or perhaps even stop using drugs altogether.

The prolonged use of recreational drugs does indeed retard progress in meditation on many fronts. Taoists in southwestern and western China have always been familiar with all forms of cannabis, as they have lived and live now in regions bordered by Laos, Vietnam, and Pakistan. They found that these substances damage the kidneys and liver and lodge resin residues in the bones of the forehead, residues that slowly leach into the brain, with undesirable results. These side effects distort the energy of the body, slowing the energetic interactions of body, chi, and spirit, which are essential to the Taoist meditation process. Some hallucinogens appear to damage brain functions, a serious obstacle to achieving internal clarity for the meditator, as well as a detriment to obtaining meditative visions, which are clouded by these drugs.

The preparatory practices of meditation can, to some degree, help the alcoholic, the abuser of drugs, and the addict. Throughout history, many chi gung and tai chi masters who practiced long hours daily were alcoholics or opium addicts. Nonetheless, they still managed to retain exceptionally high performance into old age. Normally, alcoholism and addiction to opiates weakens and destroys the body. However, the counterbalancing force of chi practices enabled these chi adepts to withstand the ravages of the toxins they had ingested. Consequently, while still feeling all the anguish that comes from addiction, these masters managed to minimize the damage done to the body through their practices.

The Taoists view addicts as people whose inner worlds are acutely uncomfortable and who take drugs to ease or avoid gnawing psychic or psychological pain. If a person who uses drugs begins to glimpse Consciousness itself, which is part of a meditator's normal spiritual growth curve, a new and satisfying internal environment may take hold. The sense of well-being and wonder at experiencing

Consciousness itself may make the effect of drugs pale by comparison. In its pure form, Taoist water method meditation or any other authentic spiritual practice may get a human being higher than any drug.* All that is required is generous portions of patience and practice.

4. Does the water method affect one's dreams?

Possibly. There seem to be two basic types of dreams. The first continues or completes internal or external events that occur during the day. The second type involves premonitions of future events, which often but not always come to pass.**

Many things affect the body, mind, and spirit during the course of a day. Most get resolved, some do not. The mind continues to process everything—feelings, perceptions, projections—always seeking resolutions. The problems you may be working on, your hopes, fears, and alternatives, are all played out in dreams. Whole schools of psychological thought attempt to interpret these dreams; whether they are successful or not is a matter of varying opinion.

When meditators practice the inner dissolving meditations, they may release memories deeply buried at the energetic level. In sleep, these memories frequently surface as dreams. The dream itself may resolve the memories or possibly just keep the internal pressure going, so that when you meditate the next day, you can delve into the essence of the dream at a much faster speed and attain resolution earlier than if the dreams had not occurred. Often when memories, including those of "past lives," are released from one's psychic body, the dreams themselves can be particularly

---

*Drug addiction experts and therapists may want to explore the possible use of Taoist meditation's inner and outer disolving practices as an adjunct therapy within a complete rehabilitation program to help individuals overcome the emotional and mental causes of drug addiction.

**Although part of some Taoist fire traditions, the water school does not have an active tradition of lucid dreaming or of being taught in dreams by noncorporeal teachers.

vivid, either in color or black and white. These dreams will often indicate normally ignored avenues that you need to work on in your future meditations.

Predictive dreams are more rare. When practitioners work with the psychic and causal bodies, intentionally or not, they may when dreaming see visions of the future. If the tie is to the causal level, the dreams will be very specific and not vague, whereas symbolic visions are usually generated at the emotional or psychic level.

Liu Hung Chieh was not someone who regularly remembered his dreams. The four vivid dreams he did recall, however, were all predictive. For example, he dreamed clearly the night before he was to take a river cruise on the Yangtse River not to get on a ship. He didn't. Shortly there-after, the ship sank, killing all on board. Liu did not normally consent to seriously teach students. The only reason he taught me was that on two separate occasions, years apart, he dreamed that he should teach a foreigner who resembled me. On each occasion, without notice, I arrived on his doorstep within the week.

Often, those who do not normally dream will, while sitting and meditating with their eyes open or closed, have visions made of the same stuff of dreams. From the Taoist meditation perspective, as well as those of many other traditions, there exists a continuum between waking reality and the dream state, making it hard to say what is real and what is a dream. A famous story from Chuang Tse concerns a man wondering if an experience was a dream or reality. He muses, "Was I a man dreaming I was a butterfly, or am I a butterfly dreaming I am a man?"

5. *Are blockages in the physical body necessarily manifested in the chi and emotional bodies?*

Blockages in the physical body are usually reflected in the chi body, but may or may not be manifested in the emotional or other higher bodies. The power that causes your physical body to work is your chi body. A distortion in your physical body will cause some distortion in your chi body, but not necessarily of equal magnitude. The distortion in your physical body could be small and its counterpart in your chi body large, or vice versa.

All this influence is based on the hierarchy of energetic relationships governing the eight bodies (see Chapter 2). The blockages or charges in the next higher body or bodies always move downward to affect the lower bodies. In contrast, any lower body has a much more restricted ability to affect the bodies above it. In general, two energetic bodies that border each other (for example, physical-chi, emotional-mental, psychic-causal) are directly linked.

What is influencing what and to what extent, however, is not always so easy to determine. The energy of a blockage as it moves upward from a lower body will always have effect on the next higher body to some extent, but it will often have little or no effect two or three bodies above. Therefore, disturbance in the physical body may or may not affect the emotional body, and the emotional body may or may not affect the higher causal body, but the emotional body will definitely influence the mental body, and the yet higher psychic body will most definitely affect all bodies below it (mental, emotional, chi, and physical bodies).

Getting a physical bruise will affect your energy body, but may not create a blockage in your emotions or intellectual processes. But a serious blockage in your emotions or way of thinking will sooner or later affect your physical body.

6. *What is the difference between quiet chi and agitated chi?*

Quiet chi has a sense of smoothness that, when experienced, takes the individual ever more strongly into stillness. Agitated chi vibrates, often very strongly, in a discomforting manner that feels outright wrong, or at the very least not quite right, to people without their knowing why. Agitated chi is one of the overt sources of the "monkey mind." The experience of the sensations of agitated chi may be subtle or rough.

7. How does the 70 percent rule apply to the mind and meditation?

Several common Western maxims carry some of the basic flavor of the 70 percent rule: "moderation in all things," "be gentle with yourself," "appreciate the fact that you have human limitations as well as possibilities," "common sense is good sense," "Rome was not built in a day," and so on.

Some of the attitudes that will cause you to violate the 70 percent rule in meditation are: "self-torture is necessary for spiritual growth," "no pain, no gain," "be perfect or die trying," "grin and bear it even though you know in your heart of hearts that you are going over the edge and will get hurt." While these attitudes prevail in most of the world's fire traditions, including those of Taoism, they are not the Taoist water method tradition.

You may have certain expectations about meditation based on what you have read or heard. It is not necessary to pressure yourself. You have to find your own balance point, one that prevents you from psychologically beating yourself up because you feel you are not progressing fast enough. Try to achieve a realistic sense of self-confidence. Don't push too hard and don't be too lazy. In meditation, people exceed the 70 percent rule when they try to be more than human. Gods may be perfect, but not humans. If you are pressuring yourself to be perfect, you most probably are about to throw the 70 percent rule out the window. In meditation, the natural desire to transform yourself spiritually is a good thing. However, this positive desire must be tempered by moderation and an acceptance that going beyond your limits, or forsaking moderation, will prevent you from reaching your goal.

When people first start meditating, going inside themselves, they often have unrealistic expectations of how much sustained pressure their nervous systems and underlying emotions can handle. Consequently, those meditators who push the envelope can destabilize, or "melt down." In regular life, the school of hard knocks trains most of us to recognize the signs that we are beginning to go over the edge. Such signs include agitation unconnected to any present life event, emotional responses that are out of proportion to simple situations, and a pervading sense of physical uneasiness when alone. If signals like these start popping up in your meditation practice, chances are good that they mean the same thing they ordinarily do: you are approaching or going over the edge. The solution: ease off, practice less, or stop for a while. If emotions are arising inside you that you do not know how to handle, slow down. It also may be a good idea to seek temporary support from a qualified professional who may have some good advice, or ask a meditation master for insights.

8. *How often do I have to keep dissolving before it really works? Twice a day? What do you suggest?*

"Before it really works?" This is similar to two virtually unanswerable questions commonly posed by neophyte meditators, namely: "How long will it take me to become spiritual?" and "How long will it take me to become enlightened?" Any individual's ability to progress in any form of meditation depends strongly on your particular karmic makeup and on the kind and quantity of internal obstacles present. Progress in meditation is not linked directly to time spent in practice. What can be said is that if some work is not done on your internal obstacles, they will remain.

When people buy a product—goods or a service—they have a reasonable right to query what expectations the product is going to fulfill, in what period of time. But meditation is not a product. However much or little you practice, it only gives you an opportunity to gain access to yourself—it does not give a guarantee. Practicing sometimes is better than not practicing at all; practicing regularly every day is better than practicing irregularly; practicing twice a day gives you more access than practicing once a day. Sometimes taking a few days or weeks alone or in a group as a meditation retreat, away from the distractions of worldly life, is also very good. In the great meditation traditions of the world, many have been known to take retreats that last for years on end.

9. Does the ability to dissolve diminish with age?

No. Usually the ability to dissolve increases with experience. In Taoism, the dissolving process is taken up quite actively by people fifty or sixty or older.

10. What should the sequence of dissolving be? Do I have to start at the top of my head and always work down, or can I begin at my kneecap and work down from there?

Beginners should always work downward only, and they should start scanning with awareness either at the top of the head or above the head at the boundary of the etheric body. Let's say you have begun moving downward and have reached your chest. If for some reason you now decide to move higher up your body (to your forehead, perhaps) because something is especially bothering you, you must redissolve again everything from your forehead to your chest before redissolving lower down your body toward either your lower tantien or feet.

Do not begin your dissolving below your head, even though the offending energy to which your mind is drawn may be located lower down your body (in your knee, for instance). Clearing what is above the main discomforting blockage, then the blockage itself, and then what is below it is required to release the blockage fully. Often when you are dissolving below your head, the source of the problem will have been resolved before you reach your knee, and when you get to your knee, the initially felt blockage is gone and no longer can be felt. This is similar to acupuncture, where putting a needle in the ear can relieve a kidney problem, whereas putting a needle at the kidney alone may not relieve the organ at all. Similarly, any problem you encounter in your body may not be completely resolved until your awareness reaches your feet, or the end of your etheric body below your feet. The energetic matrix of the human body is like a hologram, where all the parts are directly linked to some degree or another. Even for an adept, trying to second-guess differing levels of energetic primacy is difficult. The methodology of the downward-dissolving process was designed to cover all contingencies.

11. Can dissolving occur automatically without my will being involved?

Yes. In the Christian tradition, this is called grace. Grace occurs all on its own without human intervention. Usually, for the beginning meditator the will, or conscious intent, must first be used. After significant experience, rather than after philosophical musings or mere casual experience, the need to use the conscious will can be progressively replaced by a willingness to let things go when you perceive their time has past. If you can't yet let go effortlessly, using intent during the dissolving process will still be necessary.

12. Will inner and outer dissolving work for men and women equally?

Yes. There are natural differences between men and women, of course. Consequently, the genders will initially be drawn to dissolving different aspects of their internal environment. Each sex will find some things easier or more difficult to dissolve than others.

13. Can I dissolve an upper and lower spot simultaneously?

This practice is definitely not recommended for beginners. *Only the downward-dissolving practice is advised for beginners.* Simultaneously dissolving two spots is a fairly advanced practice that requires significant familiarity with the mindstream, which forms the linkage between your mundane conscious awareness and Consciousness itself. Other more advanced dissolving practices include dissolving upward, simultaneously inward and outward, center to periphery, and between entities.

14. Is there a difference between dissolving an emotion or anything else or deciding to ignore it by the force of will?

Yes. Ignoring, suppressing, and dissolving an emotion are entirely different things. As children having to mature into adults needing reasonably harmonious social interactions, we all need to learn some basic emotional self-control. Without it, we would all rip each other's throats out psychologically or physically, without reflecting on it.

However, after you move beyond this basic need for self-control, there is a major difference between ignoring or suppressing a deeply embedded emotion and resolving it. The purpose of the dissolving process is to dissolve and resolve, cut the root of the problem, and finish it, not merely to control it or allow yourself to feel better about it. You must gradually reduce the bound energy until its root is resolved, layer by layer, into Consciousness itself.

When you simply ignore or suppress an emotion, its energy is held in your mind/body and festers, sometimes gradually building to an explosive force, much like the pressure gathering in a volcano before it blows. The buildup is often extremely uncomfortable to live with, both for yourself and others. The dissolving process seeks to release the pressure a little at a time until the blocked emotional energies are dissolved back into their original source, Consciousness itself.

15. Can I use the dissolving process to get rid of things on my skin like warts and blemishes, or deeper internal problems?

I don't know. I can't say I have ever seen anyone try. However, one of my students from Britain relayed to me an interesting incident involving the dissolving experience and his skin. One summer he stepped on a wasp's nest, which shook him up. The angry wasps swarmed and stung him all over his body. He then began to dissolve where he felt the pain most intensely, deciding not to dissolve his calves, which did not feel as bad. Within several hours the considerable physical pain had vanished, and he was calm, no longer emotionally agitated. The next day, the only place in his body that had any pain from the stings were his calves, which he did not dissolve.

In China for thousands of years both chi gung and Taoist meditation also used the dissolving process to heal serious problems inside the body. Once a pregnant student asked me if fibroids could be dissolved, as during her first trimester she developed an extremely large set of fibroids, which were currently growing. After tests the doctors told her that the fibroids had already developed into a large solid mass that would definitely block the birth canal, making a caesarean section necessary. She wanted a natural birth. I said that during my time in China gynecological problems were not my focus as a chi gung therapist, and as such I had no direct experience with fibroids. However, diligent use of the dissolving process has been known to work with other physical problems. I suggested she try, but I offered no guarantees.

She tried. Several months later her hard work paid off. Tests showed that the fibroids had liquefied sufficiently to allow a natural birth. As fate would have it, however, she ended up having a caesarean birth anyway—not because of the fibroids, but because the baby was in breech position. She is currently the mother of a healthy baby girl.

16. Can the dissolving process be done while I have earphones on listening to music?

For the beginner, no. In the beginning especially, your undivided attention is absolutely required. Once you become adept at it, you should be equally able to dissolve in the middle of the most horrific or pleasurable situation or noise. Of course, many forms of music are relaxing and emotionally uplifting. Music can take you out of yourself and the incessant problems of life. If you want to go deeper inside yourself and find Consciousness, however, silence is a better complement to meditation than music. Although both music and meditation can tend to put you into a more satisfying emotional space, meditation will eventually enable you to get directly to the heart space without any external vehicles, such as music, art, or other people.

17. Is there any advantage to dissolving in one modality over the other?

Not really. The five modes simply include all the situations life will put you in: that is, standing, moving, sitting, lying down, and during sex. Whether one part of life is more advantageous, is better or worse, than another is a matter of personal philosophy. What can be said is that some modalities are easier than others for learning the dissolving process. The outer dissolving process is most easily learned standing. The inner dissolving process is most easily learned sitting. The most difficult way to learn both inner and outer dissolving is lying down.

Energy Anatomy of the Human Body

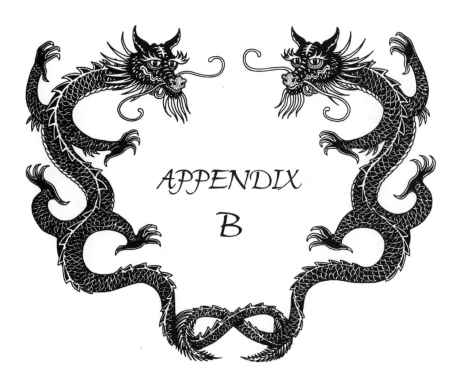

APPENDIX

B

Reprinted from *The Power of Internal Martial Arts*

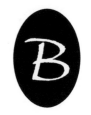

Energy Anatomy of the Human Body

The Main Energy Channels and the Three Tantiens

What Is Common to the Left, Right, and Central Energy Channels

Three main energy channels, or paths of flow—the left, right, and central channels (see Figures 1 and 2)—begin at conception and remain within a person throughout life. Other important energies move in the human body according to meridian patterns that have been well mapped by Chinese medicine. Any text on acupuncture should include charts that identify them. The left, right, and central channels, however, according to Taoist chi gung theory, come into existence before the acupuncture meridians and create these meridians during fetal evelopment. The three main energy channels have certain characteristics in common.

All three, for example, are located in the center of the body; that is, in each, the energy flows occur midway between the skin in the front of the body and the skin in the back of the body.

Also, the central channel joins the right channel on the right side of the body and the left channel on the left side at the tips of the fingers, the tips of the toes, the center of the armpits, kwa, and at the *ba hui* point, which is located on the center of the crown of the head.

The Pathway of the Central Channel

In the torso and head: The central channel runs from the center of the perineum (the area between the anus and the posterior part of the external genitalia) through the center of the torso to the bai hui point on the center of the crown of the head. The channel runs through internal organs, soft tissues, blood vessels, and the brain.

In the arms: The central channel runs from the heart center (middle tantien) to a meeting point in the center of the armpits, where the energies of the central and left or right channels temporarily join. From the armpits, the energy of the central channel moves through the bone marrow of the arm bones, through the center of the elbows and then the wrist joints to the center of the palms and from there, via the bone marrow, to the fingertips. In the fingertips, the energies of the right and left channels on their respective sides merge with the energy of the central channel and, once joined, continue to the edge of the etheric body.

In the legs: The central channel runs through the bone marrow from the perineum between the legs along a line continuing across the pelvis to the kwa and hip sockets. From there it travels through the bone marrow of the leg bones, through the knee and ankle joints, then through the center of each foot along a midline from the heel to the ball of the foot and then through the bone marrow of the toes.

Where the central channel exits the body: The energy of the central channel mingles with the energies of the right and left channels and the commingled energies exit from the physical body to the etheric body at these points:

1. From the end of the fingertips and the tips of the toes, extending to the boundary of the etheric body.

2. From the bai hui point at the crown of the head to the boundary of the etheric body above the head, where one's own personal energy connects with the energy of heaven (cosmic energy).

3. From the center of the ball of each foot extending out to below the feet, to the boundary of the etheric body beneath, where one's personal energy connects with the energy of the earth.

Figure 1: The Central Channel

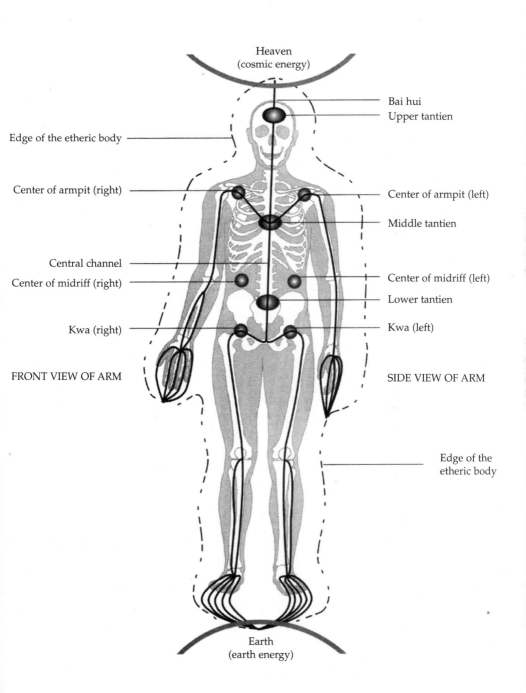

Heaven
(cosmic energy)

Bai hui
Upper tantien

Edge of the etheric body

Center of armpit (right)

Center of armpit (left)

Middle tantien

Central channel
Center of midriff (right)

Center of midriff (left)

Lower tantien

Kwa (right)

Kwa (left)

FRONT VIEW OF ARM

SIDE VIEW OF ARM

Edge of the
etheric body

Earth
(earth energy)

The Pathway of the Left and Right Channels

In the head and shoulders: From the crown of the head down to the collarbone, at no time do the left and right channels intersect the central channel. The left and right channels begin at the bai hui point at the crown of the head (where their energies are merged with that of the central channel). They continue down the center of the brain going parallel on either side of the central channel at an imperceptible distance away from it. At the upper tantien (third eye), the distance between the left and right channels widens, and they continue down to the center of the eyes, to the nostrils, down each side of the mouth, down the throat, to the level of the clavicals, close to but without intersecting the central channel. At this point the left and right channels branch off on a line to the left and to the right along the center line between the clavicals and back, where they join temporarily with the central channel in the center of the armpits, before splitting off again.

In the arms: From the center of the armpits on their respective sides of the body, the left and right channels run down each arm to the fingertips within the bone matrix (calicum) of both the bones of the arm and the joints to the ends of the five fingertips. Here, the left and right channels merge with the central channel.

In the legs: Beginning from the kwa (inguinal fold), both the left and right channels run within the bone matrix of their respective hip sockets, thigh and shin bones, knee and ankle joints, within the small bones of the feet along two thin parallel lines on either side of the central channel, to the center of the ball of the foot where the left right and central channels merge. They then split again and go to the tips of the toes, where again the left and right channels merge with the central channel and the commingled energy continues to the boundary of the etheric body.

The control gates of the left and right channels: There are three energetic "sluice gates" that either allow energy to pass unimpeded through the left and right channels or diminish it or completely cut off its flow. These are located in the center of the armpits, the center of the midriff, and the kwa.

Figure 2: The Left and Right Channels

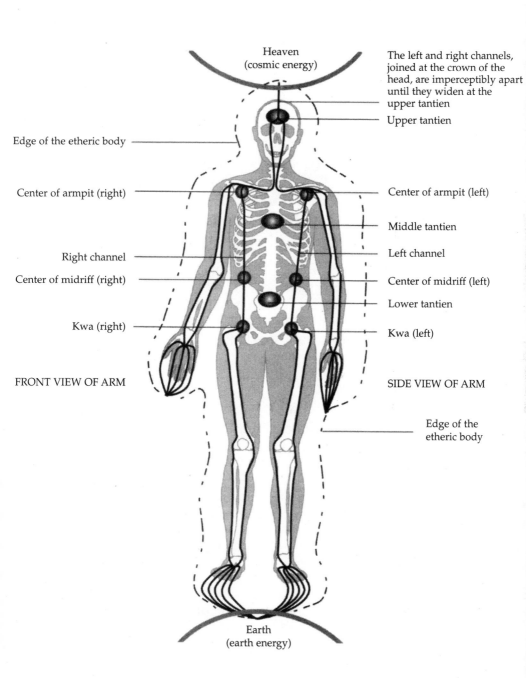

Heaven
(cosmic energy)

The left and right channels, joined at the crown of the head, are imperceptibly apart until they widen at the upper tantien

Upper tantien

Edge of the etheric body

Center of armpit (right)

Center of armpit (left)

Middle tantien

Right channel

Left channel

Center of midriff (right)

Center of midriff (left)

Lower tantien

Kwa (right)

Kwa (left)

FRONT VIEW OF ARM

SIDE VIEW OF ARM

Edge of the etheric body

Earth
(earth energy)

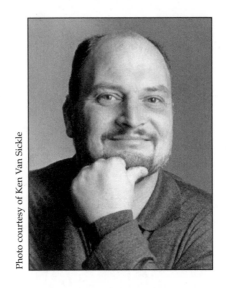

Bruce Kumar Frantzis, lineage master in the Taoist arts, has been working since 1961 in Eastern healing systems, chi gung, martial arts and meditation, including sixteen years in Japan, India and China. He spent twenty years studying Zen, Yoga, Kundalini and Taoist Fire traditions. This training provided the foundation for extensive study of the Water Method with Taoist Lineage Master Liu Hung Chieh in Beijing, China.

B. K. Frantzis is the founder of Energy Arts, Inc., based in Marin County, California. Energy Arts offers instructor certification programs, retreats and corporate and public seminars in North America and Europe. Frantzis teaches Energy Arts courses in meditation, breathing, chi gung, tai chi, ba gua, hsing-i and related subjects.

For details of events, instructional materials and certified instructors, visit the Energy Arts website, www.energyarts.com

A 2–CD set, *Taoist Breathing*, is available as a companion to this Water Meditation series.

Energy Arts, Inc.
P. O. Box 99, Fairfax, CA 94978
(415) 454-5243   (415) 454-0907 fax
www.energyarts.com